indian
Recipes and Home Remedies

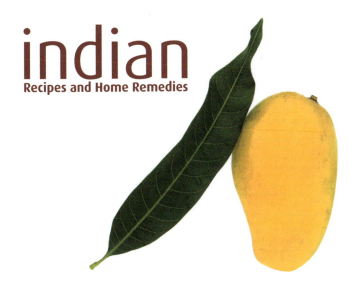

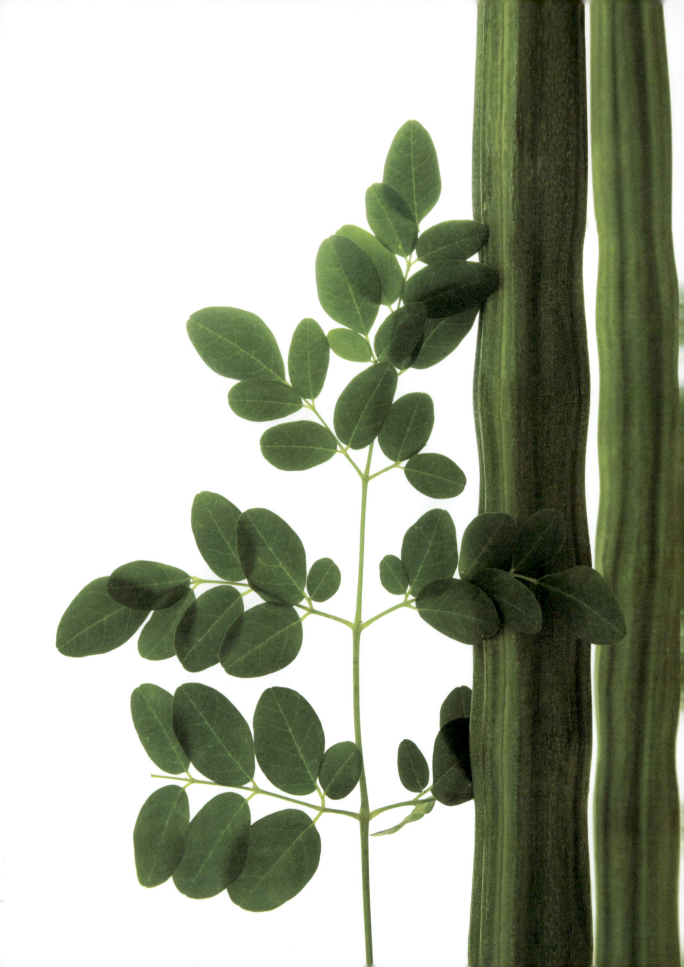

naturally speaking
indian
Recipes and Home Remedies

Devagi Sanmugam

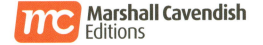

Marshall Cavendish
Editions

Design : Lynn Chin Nyuk Ling
Photography : Joshua Tan, Elements by the Box

© 2007 Marshall Cavendish International (Asia) Private Limited

Published by Marshall Cavendish Editions
An imprint of Marshall Cavendish International
1 New Industrial Road, Singapore 536196

This publication represents the opinions and views of the author based on her personal experience, knowledge and research. The information in this book is not intended for use in place of proper medical advice. Persons with medical conditions should consult qualified physicians before starting any form of treatment. The author and publisher have used their best efforts in preparing this book and disclaim liability rising directly and indirectly from the use and application of this book.

Other Marshall Cavendish Offices:
Marshall Cavendish Ltd. 119 Wardour Street, London W1F 0UW, UK • Marshall Cavendish Corporation. 99 White Plains Road, Tarrytown NY 10591-9001, USA • Marshall Cavendish International (Thailand) Co Ltd. 253 Asoke, 12th Flr, Sukhumvit 21 Road, Klongtoey Nua, Wattana, Bangkok 10110, Thailand • Marshall Cavendish (Malaysia) Sdn Bhd, Times Subang, Lot 46, Subang Hi-Tech Industrial Park, Batu Tiga, 40000 Shah Alam, Selangor Darul Ehsan, Malaysia

Marshall Cavendish is a trademark of Times Publishing Limited.

National Library Board Singapore Cataloguing in Publication Data

Devagi Sanmugam.
Naturally speaking : Indian recipes and home remedies / Devagi Sanmugam. – Singapore : Marshall Cavendish Editions, 2007.
p. cm.
ISBN-13 : 978-981-232-715-4
ISBN-10 : 981-232-715-0

1. Traditional medicine – India. 2. Functional foods – India. 3. Medicine, Ayurvedic. 4. Indian cookery. I. Title.

TX724.5.I4
641.5954 -- dc22   SLS2006053171

Printed in China by Everbest Printing Co Ltd

Acknowledgements

I would like to thank the following persons for their help in gathering the material for this book: Sujatha, Kannan, Pravin, Pushpa Rajoo, Indhumathy, Komala Gunabalan, Bavani, Anjalai Markandan, Kalyani, Dinesh, Makeasan, Aravind, Velavan, Devarajan, Prateep, Sulochana, Devagi Janasegaran, Hitesh, Sivaraman, Sivakumar, Manogaran, Ramachandra M K and Muruganandan.

I also wish to dedicate this book to my husband, Shanmugam, and all those who have never had grandmothers to prepare home remedies for them!

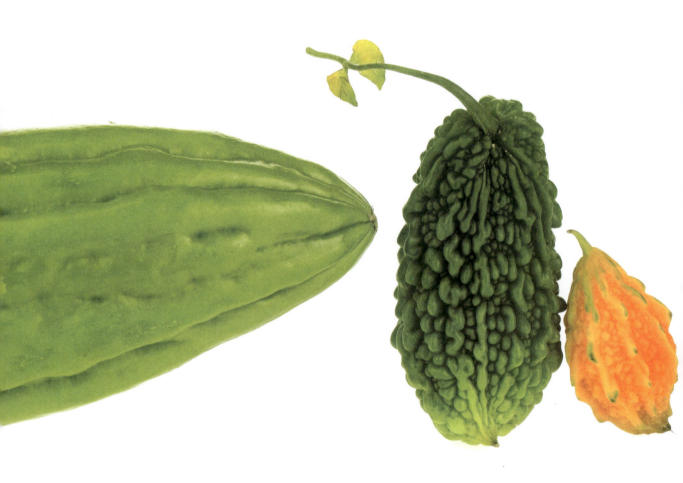

Foreword

In the days before western medicine became widely practised, many Indian women in Singapore had a good knowledge of home remedies and recipes made with a wide variety of herbs and spices commonly found in the home, to treat all sorts of ailments and to maintain good health. My grandmother and mother were among them. Many spices commonly found in the stock cupboard such as ajwain and cumin were used to treat bouts of indigestion; a plant or fruit planted in the home compound could also be plucked, as and when required for some form of beauty treatment or remedy to be had.

When I was growing up, a coconut or gingelly oil massage for the whole body before a bath was a weekly ritual to promote good circulation while a drink of ajwain water after a heavy meal (especially one that included a mutton dish) to aid digestion was a must. Eating Indian gooseberries for good health was also encouraged whenever the extremely sour fruit was in season. For relieving nausea and treating diarrhoea, my grandmother prescribed a brew of black tea without any sugar or milk — a handy treatment which I still follow today. Turmeric was my grandmother's favourite spice for treating stomach upsets; a teaspoonful of turmeric powder stirred in a glass of warm water and drunk, works wonders.

All these natural home remedies and recipes advocated by the older generation are treatments which, I think, have kept them healthy, active and energetic well into old age. I feel really lucky to have a grandmother and mother who have shown me all these natural remedies and recipes for everyday health and living. As the common saying goes, 'Good health is the greatest wealth of mankind'. In this book, I would like to share with you the same remedies and recipes for a healthy living.

Most of the ingredients featured in this book are herbs and spices including various plants, fruits, vegetables and seeds. I have, however, included a few non-herb items, namely, ghee, jaggery and honey for two reasons; they are essential items in any Indian pantry cupboard and also provide an impressive repertoire of healing properties and treatments for the home.

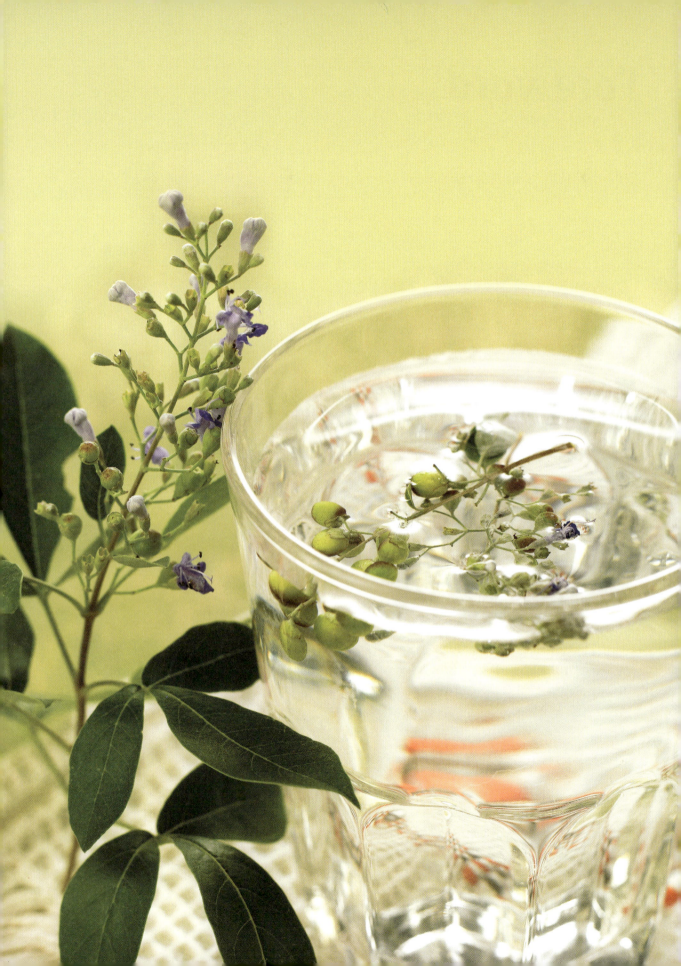

Introduction

The Principles of Ayurveda

Any discussion of natural Indian healing traditions will include a mention of Ayurveda, which means "the science of life" in Sanskrit. Ayurveda is an ancient science of healing which can be traced back to the ancient Vedic culture in India more than 5,000 years ago. It is an all-encompassing healing system which encourages the maintenance of good health and the prevention of diseases by creating the right balance in one's body, mind and spirit. This balance is managed via correct thinking, lifestyle, diet and the use of herbs, of which herbal remedies are discussed in this book.

According to Ayurveda, food forms our best medicinal treatments as 'we are what we eat'. Everything that we consume, including herbs and spices, can be classified according to the 'six tastes' approach: sweet, sour, salty, pungent, bitter and astringent; each 'taste' carries out a specific bodily function. Foods with a 'sweet taste' are nutritious for the body and help build body tissue; they are sources of carbohydrates, fats and proteins which include honey, milk, breads and meats. The 'sour taste' is derived from foods with natural organic acids such as citrus fruits, pickles and tomatoes, which stimulate appetite and also improve digestion. The 'salty flavour' is obtained from sources such as salt, salted meats and sauces; salty foods serve as mild laxatives and sedatives, and promote digestion. Pungent foods include onions, garlic and pepper. They help stimulate digestion and clear congestion. Bitter foods include leafy greens, coriander and fenugreek and are anti-inflammatory and detoxifying for the body. Foods with astringent properties include apples, pomegranates and tea. These are diuretic and detoxify the body as well as improve blood circulation. To eat healthily, it is essential that all the 'six tastes' are present at every meal. Various herbs and spices are thus important ingredients for cooking dishes which are appetising as well as easily digestible.

The Five Primary Elements

According to Ayurvedic philosophy, the entire cosmos is organised according to five primary elements which are:

SPACE the unified field in which all forces of nature are expressed and the source of all other elements.

AIR the motion principle which guides the flow of energy in all living systems.

FIRE the principle of metabolism and transformation which guides the production of energy in stars and the cells of the human body alike.

WATER the principle of cohesive forces, ranging from the gravitational pull of planets to its role as a life source in which biological systems evolve.

EARTH the principle which governs the existence of physical matter such as planets, bodies and cells.

The Three Principal Energies of the Body: Vata, Pitta and Kapha

According to Ayurveda, the five elements described above can be further reduced to three principal energies, namely, Vata, Pitta and Kapha. These determine our mind-body constitutions.

VATA Composed of a mixture of Space and Air elements, Vata is the energy of movement which oversees bodily functions such as breathing, muscle and tissue movement as well as the beating of the heart. When Vata is aggravated, we suffer from anxiety, excessive flatulence, and heart palpitations; this energy can be restored to balance by taking calming herbs, foods and meditation.

PITTA Comprising Fire and Water elements, Pitta is the energy of metabolism which affects digestion, the absorption of nutrients and body temperature. When Pitta is out of balance, we experience heartburn, skin rashes, the inflammation of organs and irritability. 'Cooling' herbs are beneficial in relieving Pitta-aggravated conditions.

KAPHA The third principal energy, Kapha, a combination of Earth and Water elements, is responsible for holding our physical framework of bones, muscles and tendons together and providing fluid lubrication for our skins and joints. When Kapha is out of balance, water retention and sinus can occur; herbs and spices that are 'heaty' and aromatic are useful for restoring balance to the body system.

In essence, it is believed in Ayurveda that all human beings possess a predominant mind-body constitution which determines their physical and physiological characteristics as well as personalities. For example, Pitta-dominant persons are said to have warm bodies, with medium-sized body frames and a short temper.

It appears then, that in its strictest form, when prescribing herbal remedies for various treatments according to Ayurvedic traditions, a combination of factors including the inherent tastes of the food (is it sweet, sour, bitter, pungent, salty or astringent?), the nature of the illness (is it a phelgmy or dry cough?) as well as the innate mind-body constitution of the sick person (is he or she a Vata-dominant, Pitta-dominant or Kapha-dominant type?) have to be taken into account to offer the most effective form of treatment for the patient.

However, it should be noted that the discussion of herbal treatments, according to the strictest traditions of Ayurvedic medicine are beyond the scope of this book, which focuses on simple remedies, recipes and beauty treatments for everyday healthy living. Unless otherwise specified, the dosages or applications prescribed in the remedies of this book are for a single person. For illnesses of a serious nature and persistent ailments, or if you are unsure about taking certain remedies, please seek proper medical attention or advice from your doctor or a certified Ayurvedic practitioner.

Glossary

Throughout this book, you will come across various terms that describe the healing properties of the herbs, spices and other ingredients. The following is a useful guide for your easy reference.

ANODYNE refers to any herb or spice that acts as a natural painkiller.

AROMATIC applied mostly to scented herbs and spices, generally good for improving digestion.

ASTRINGENT associated mainly with substances that contain tannic acids. They contract, firm and strengthen skin and other tissue. Also used in the treatment of inflammation.

CARMINATIVE applied to any herb and spice which relieves flatulence and helps in treating colic.

DEMULCENT applied mostly to substances which help soothe inflamed or irritated internal tissue such as mucous membranes.

EXPECTORANT closely associated with any herbal remedy that aids coughs. It helps to loosen thick phlegm so that the phlegm can be coughed up easily.

LAXATIVE helps in the stimulation or evacuation of the bowels by softening and lubricating hard stools.

TONIC in general, it is applied to those herbs that stimulate or nourish the various organs of the body.

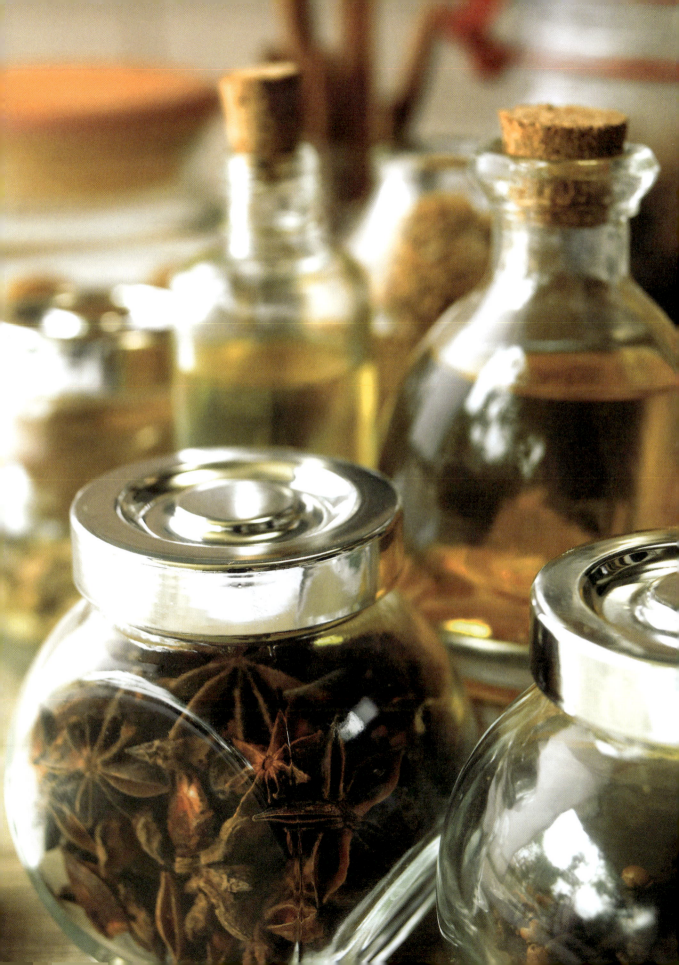

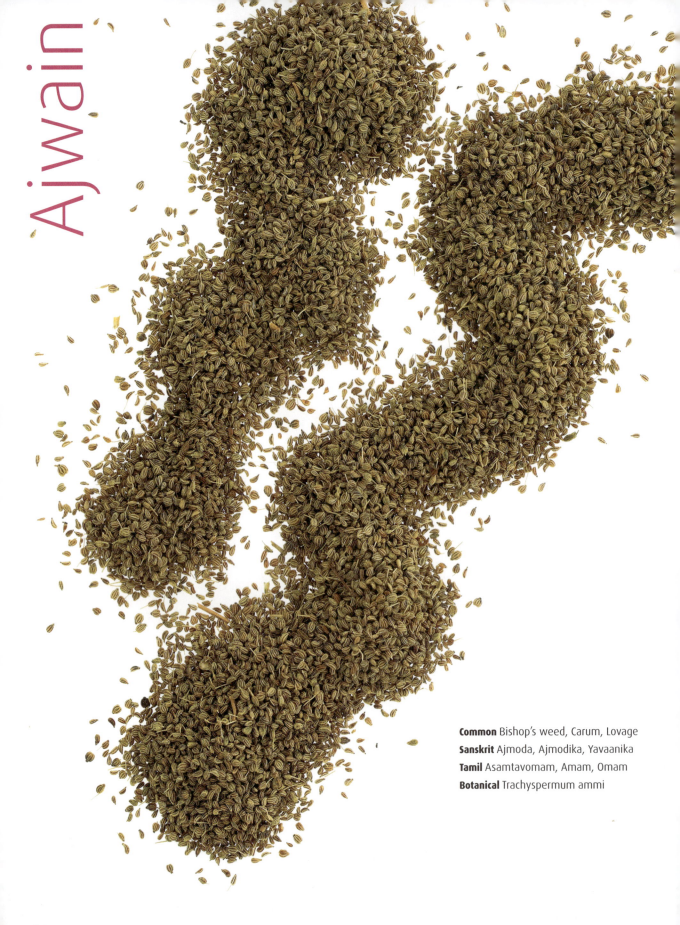

Ajwain

Common Bishop's weed, Carum, Lovage
Sanskrit Ajmoda, Ajmodika, Yavaanika
Tamil Asamtavomam, Amam, Omam
Botanical Trachyspermum ammi

Ajwain, also known as Bishop's weed is an aromatic spice with a bitter taste similar to thyme. The small, brown seeds with light-coloured stripes closely resemble cumin seeds.

Originating in the Middle East, ajwain seeds are widely grown throughout India and the seeds are often used in home remedies for stomach-related ailments such as indigestion and flatulence. It is quite common to see a bottle of distilled ajwain water in the cupboards of most South Indian homes. In fact, some grandmothers force their grandchildren to drink about one tablespoonful of distilled ajwain water to aid digestion after a heavy meal. Ajwain seeds have traces of protein, minerals, fibre, carbohydrates, calcium, phosphorus, iron, carotene, thiamin, riboflavin and niacin.

They are an integral part of the Indian kitchen and are often used for their aromatic flavour in a wide variety of food such as pickles, savoury snacks, breads and pastries. Ajwain seeds also act as a carminative to counteract the effects of ingredients such as lentils, pulses and wheat flour that may cause indigestion and flatulence. Ground ajwain seeds can also be mixed with water and used as a fungicide on organic plants.

Remedy for Nasal Congestion

Turmeric powder $1/4$ tsp
Ajwain seeds 1 tsp, lightly crushed
Water 250 ml (8 fl oz/ 1 cup)

Boil all ingredients together for 3 minutes and inhale the vapours for a few minutes to clear a blocked nose.

Note: You can also stir in 1 tsp honey and drink the mixture after it has cooled down, preferably before bedtime, for a better sleep.

FROM LEFT TO RIGHT: *Cauliflower Pakora (page 16), Remedy for Nasal Congestion (page 15)*

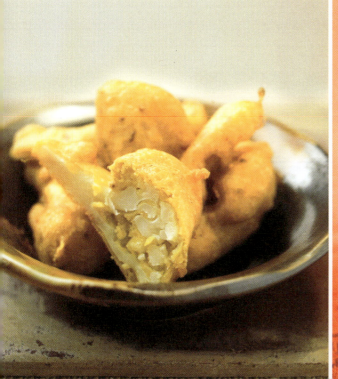
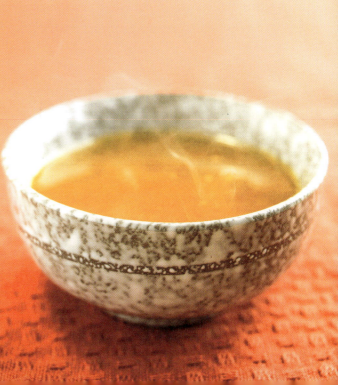

Cauliflower Pakora

Preparation time: 15 minutes
Cooking time: 15 minutes
Serves: 5

Cauliflower 750 g (1 lb 10 oz),
cut into small florets

Cooking oil for deep-frying

Batter

Chickpea flour (*besan*) 300 g (10^1/$_2$ oz)

Rice flour 30 g (1 oz)

Turmeric powder 1 tsp

Baking powder ^{1}/$_2$ tsp

Salt 1^1/$_2$ tsp

Ground ginger 1^1/$_2$ tsp

Meat curry powder 2 tsp

Ajwain seeds 1 tsp, lightly crushed

Water 250 ml (8 fl oz / 1 cup)

Put all ingredients for batter into a large mixing bowl and combine well to form a smooth batter. Set aside for 15 minutes.

Dip cauliflower florets into prepared batter. Coat well and deep-fry in hot oil until golden brown.

Drain on absorbent paper towels and serve hot as a snack.

Murukku

Ajwain seeds are an important ingredient in murukku. These seeds reduce flatulence as two types of lentil flours are used here.

Preparation time: 10 minutes
Cooking time: 15 minutes
Serves: 6

Water 300 ml (10 fl oz / 1^1/$_4$ cups)

Coconut cream 80 ml
(2^1/$_2$ fl oz / ^{1}/$_3$ cup) (see note)

Caster (superfine) sugar ^{1}/$_2$ tsp

Salt 1^1/$_4$ tsp

Ghee (clarified butter) 1 Tbsp

Rice flour 200 g (7 oz), sifted

Chickpea flour (*besan*) 50 g
(2 oz), sifted

Skinned black lentil flour (*urad* dhal flour) 100 g (3 ^{1}/$_2$ oz), sifted

Ajwain seeds 1 tsp, lightly crushed

Ground black pepper 1 tsp

Black sesame seeds 1 Tbsp

Put water, coconut cream, sugar, salt and ghee into a pan and bring to the boil. Remove from heat.

Place remaining ingredients into a mixing bowl and pour in boiled mixture. Combine well and knead to form a soft dough.

Place some dough into a murukku press and press out the dough onto a sheet of cling film (plastic wrap) or a piece of clean, damp cloth.

Deep-fry a few murukku at a time in hot oil until crisp. Drain on absorbent paper towels. Store in airtight containers when completely cooled. Serve as a light snack.

Note: To obtain coconut cream, place the freshly grated flesh of a coconut into a cheesecloth and squeeze firmly to extract the thick liquid. Use as required. For convenience, use cartons of ready-to-use coconut cream which are now available at most Asian grocery stores.

Remedy for Flatulence

Take this remedy to relieve indigestion, repeated belching and flatulence.

Ginger powder 4 tsp

Ajwain seeds 4 tsp

Black salt ^{1}/$_4$ tsp

Warm water 250 ml (8 fl oz / 1 cup)

Grind all ingredients except water into a fine powder and store in an airtight container. Powder can be kept for up to 6 months.

When required, mix 1 tsp powder in water and drink this portion once daily.

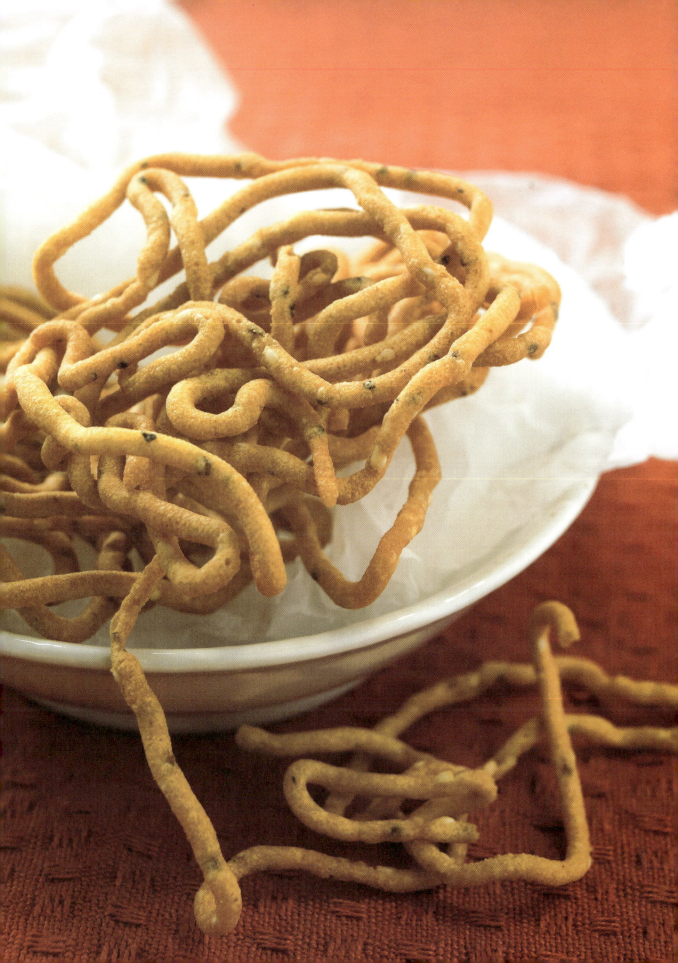

Aloe Vera

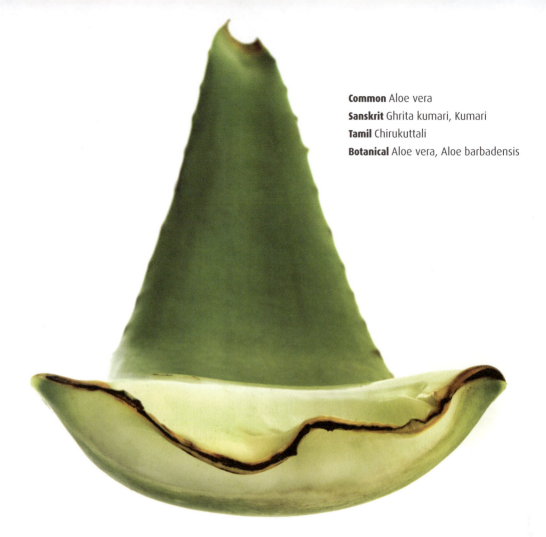

Common Aloe vera
Sanskrit Ghrita kumari, Kumari
Tamil Chirukuttali
Botanical Aloe vera, Aloe barbadensis

Throughout the centuries, the aloe vera plant has been used for a variety of medicinal purposes in India.

This healing plant has stiff grey-green, lance-shaped leaves. Each leaf comprises three layers: an outer thick skin, an inner lining and a central pulp containing clear gel. Native to southern and eastern Africa and cultivated in countries such as India and Australia, this hardy succulent contains 99 percent water. The remaining one percent is made up of chemical compounds including vitamins, minerals, enzymes and amino acids.

Many Indians regard the aloe gel as the best home remedy for treating external injuries such as minor burns, insect bites and skin irritations. Taken internally, the aloe vera gel treats ailments such as constipation, coughs, peptic ulcers, diabetes and menstrual disorders. However, when extracting aloe gel from the fresh leaf for internal use, be careful not to let the bitter juice from the inner lining of the leaf contaminate the gel as the juice has a strong laxative effect. The aloe vera gel is also commonly used in many home beauty treatments by Indian ladies for rejuvenating dry skin and improving skin tone.

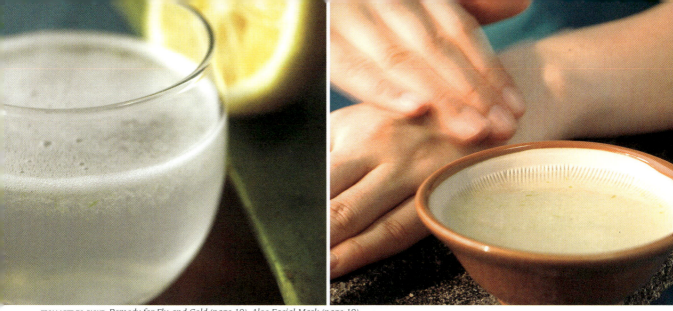

FROM LEFT TO RIGHT: Remedy for Flu and Cold (page 19), Aloe Facial Mask (page 19)

Remedy for Flu and Cold

Since aloe vera juice is good for building up the immune system, it is useful for keeping flu or a cold at bay.

Aloe vera juice 3 Tbsp
Lemon juice 1 Tbsp
Water 200 ml (6²/₃ fl oz / ³/₄ cup)

Mix all ingredients together and drink the mixture. Make and drink this portion a few times throughout the day, if desired.

Aloe Facial Mask

Try this moisturising mask to improve skin tone and achieve a smooth complexion.

Ground rice 1 Tbsp
Brown sugar 1 tsp
Aloe vera gel 2 Tbsp
Lemon juice 1 Tbsp

Combine all ingredients in a clean bowl to form a smooth paste.

Gently massage onto clean, damp skin. Leave on for 5–10 minutes.

Rinse off with warm water and pat dry with a clean towel.

Note: For a fantastic body scrub, prepare up to 4–5 times the amount of this recipe.

Aloe Mask for Oily Skin

Aloe vera gel 2 Tbsp
Lemon juice 2 Tbsp
Egg white 1

Combine aloe vera gel and lemon juice. Set aside.

Beat egg white until fluffy, then fold in aloe vera mixture. Blend well.

Apply all over face to form a thin film and leave on for 15 minutes.

Rinse off with cool water thoroughly and pat dry with a clean towel.

For sunburn, tear open an aloe plant leaf and apply the gel directly onto the affected skin. The gel has soothing and cooling, as well as antibacterial and anti-fungal properties that will help the skin heal rapidly. Some Indian women I know, also use the aloe gel to treat dandruff by applying it onto damp hair and leaving it on for 15 minutes before shampooing as per normal.

Asafoetida

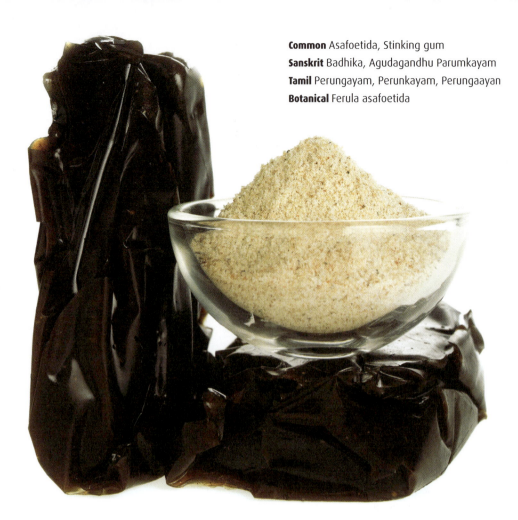

Common Asafoetida, Stinking gum
Sanskrit Badhika, Agudagandhu Parumkayam
Tamil Perungayam, Perunkayam, Perungaayan
Botanical Ferula asafoetida

Asafoetida is a resin obtained from the stem and roots of the asafoetida plant. Upon incision of the plant parts, the gum oozes out and dries into a blackish-brown coloured resin.

Most commonly used in Indian vegetarian cooking, asafoetida is often added to curries and pickles. With a flavour similar to onions and garlic, asafoetida is used as a substitute by the Brahmins and Jains in India who do not eat garlic or onions. The spice is available in solid or powdered form. In solid form, the resin is very strongly scented and should be used sparingly. It is necessary to fry the resin briefly in hot oil before cooking with it as it will then dissolve and mix well with the food. At the same time, the heat of the oil will convert the strong flavour of the spice to a more pleasant taste. To flavour a large pot of food, a pea-sized amount is considered adequate. Asafoetida powder, on the other hand, is less intense in flavour and may be added directly to the food when cooking. However, the resulting aroma will develop less deeply. While asafoetida powder is found to lose its aroma after some years, the resin appears to be unperishable and retains its flavour indefinitely.

Asafoetida is used in both Indian cooking and medicine as a carminative to treat flatulence and indigestion as well as dry coughs, asthma and heart diseases. It is said that asafoetida works as a natural insect repellent; rubbing asafoetida powder on the skin helps prevent insect bites.

Lentil Rice

Preparation time: 10 minutes
Cooking time: 15 minutes
Serves: 5

Skinned split green (mung) beans (*moong* **dhal**) 150 g (5$^1/_3$ oz)

Ghee (clarified butter) or corn oil 2 Tbsp

Black peppercorns 1$^1/_2$ Tbsp, coarsely pounded

Cumin seeds 2 tsp

Onions 2, medium, peeled and finely chopped

Ginger 2-cm knob, peeled and finely minced

Long-grain rice 500 g (1 lb 1$^1/_2$ oz), washed and well-drained

Curry powder 1 Tbsp

Water 1 litre (32 fl oz / 4 cups)

Salt 1$^1/_2$ tsp

Asafoetida powder 1 tsp

Coriander (cilantro) leaves (optional)

Dry-roast green beans until aromatic and golden brown. Cool thoroughly.

Wash and drain well. Set aside.

Heat ghee or oil and fry black peppercorns and cumin seeds until aromatic.

Add onions and ginger. Sauté until onions turn light brown.

Transfer to a rice cooker. Add remaining ingredients and mix well. Turn on rice cooker.

When rice is cooked, fluff up rice with a wooden spoon. Serve hot with a salad or vegetable. Garnish with coriander leaves, if desired.

Note: If a rice cooker is unavailable, use a deep pot. Add remaining ingredients when water boils. Mix well. Reduce heat to low, cover pot and gently simmer, stirring occasionally until rice is cooked and water has evaporated.

Blood Sugar Control Remedy

Bitter gourd juice 1 Tbsp

Asafoetida powder $^1/_4$ tsp

Mix all ingredients together and consume. Take this portion at least twice a day.

FROM LEFT TO RIGHT: *Lentil Rice (page 21), Blood Sugar Control Remedy (page 21)*

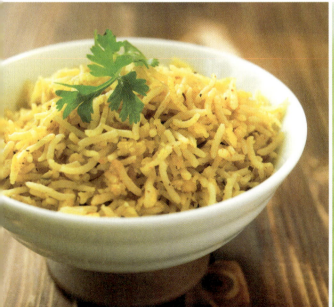
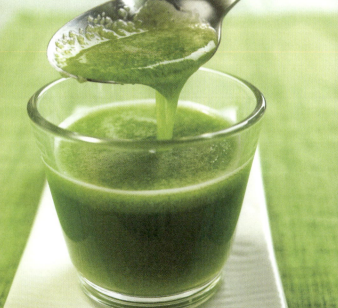

Cabbage Dhal Curry

Preparation time: 15 minutes
Cooking time: 15 minutes
Serves: 6

Skinned split green (mung) beans (*moong* **dhal)** 180 g (6 1/2 oz), washed and drained

Ghee (clarified butter) 1 tsp

Turmeric powder 1 tsp

Green chillies 3, finely chopped

Water 1.25 litres, (40 fl oz / 5 cups)

Cabbage 500 g (1 lb 1 1/2 oz), finely chopped

Salt 1 1/4 tsp

Cumin powder 2 tsp

Ghee (clarified butter) 1 Tbsp

Onion 1, peeled and thinly sliced

Asafoetida powder 1 tsp

Dry Spices

Black mustard seeds 1 tsp

Cumin seeds 1 tsp

Fennel seeds 1/2 tsp

Dried chillies 2, cut into 3-cm (1 1/2-in) pieces

Put green beans, ghee, turmeric powder, chillies and water in a large pot. Bring to the boil, then reduce heat and simmer until dhal is cooked and mushy.

Add cabbage, salt and cumin powder, then stir to mix well. Cover partially and simmer over low heat until cabbage is cooked.

In a separate pan, heat ghee and fry dry spices until aromatic and chillies turn brown.

Add onion and asafoetida powder. Sauté until onion is golden brown.

Transfer mixture to simmering dhal and cabbage mixture. Simmer for another 2 minutes, then remove from heat and serve hot with rice.

Remedy for Headaches and Menstrual Cramps

Drink this portion to relieve headaches caused by tension and menstrual cramps.

Crumbled dried asafoetida a pinch

Water 375 ml (12 fl oz / 1 1/2 cups)

Simmer all ingredients together for about 10 minutes.

Drink this portion once a day until symptoms subside.

Toothache Remedy

Asafoetida 0.5-cm (1/4-in) thick piece

Freshly squeezed lemon juice 2 Tbsp

Soak asafoetida in lemon juice and warm juice slightly until asafoetida dissolves.

Dip a piece of cotton wool in the mixture and place it in tooth cavity for quick relief.

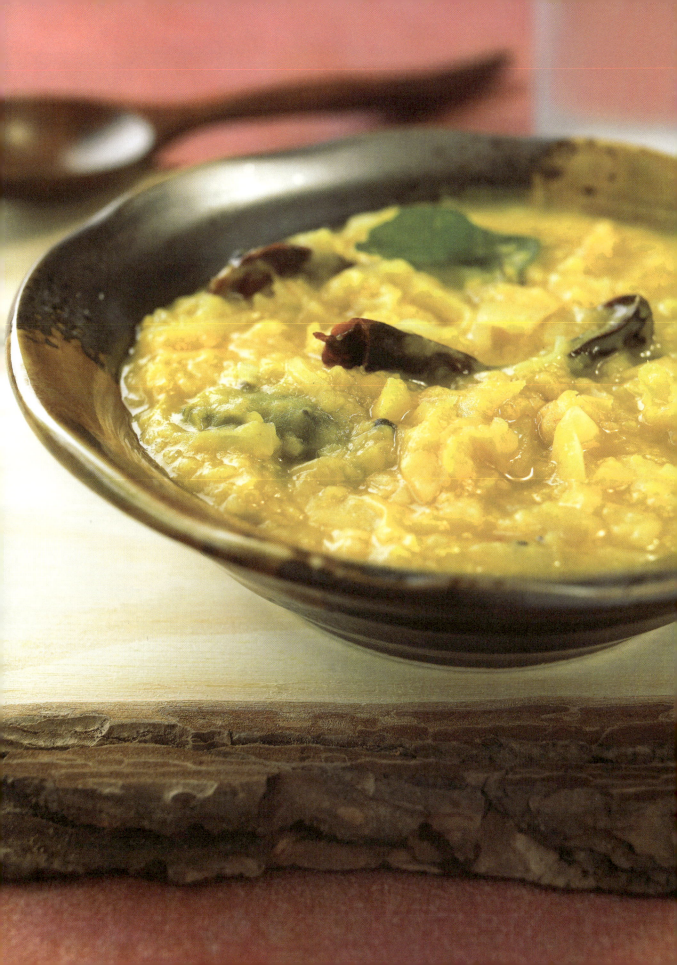

Banana

Common Banana, Plantain (cooking banana)

Sanskrit Kadli (banana), Kadali (plantain)

Tamil Vazha, Vaazhaipazham (bananas), Vaazhaikaai (plantain)

Botanical Musa paradisiaca

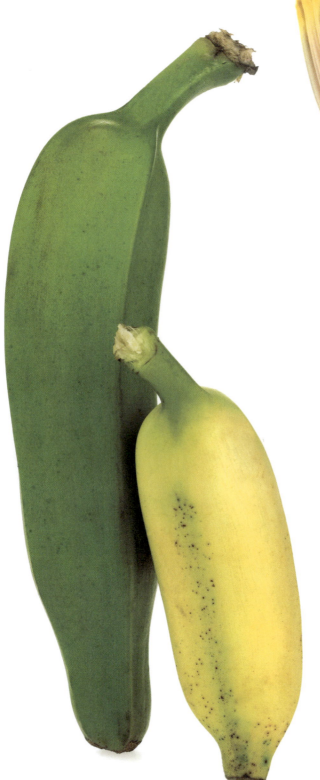

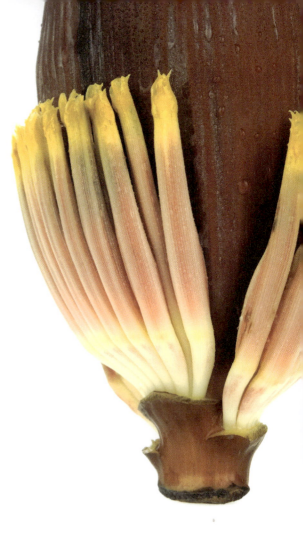

An important fruit crop in India, the banana is rich in carbohydrates and minerals such as calcium, potassium, iron and phosphorous. Bananas are highly nutritious, palatable and easily digestible, and thus are great for regulating the bowel movement, curing both constipation and diarrhoea.

In India, it is a common practice to peel and cut ripe bananas into thin slices which are then sun-dried and ground into a fine powder for babies. The powder is boiled with milk and a pinch of salt until thickened. The mixture is fed to babies who are beginning to take semi-solid foods. This nutritious and easily digestible concoction is believed to prevent diarrhoea as well as worm infection in babies.

Enclosed within the long, oval and purple-coloured banana flower bud are small, pinkish and yellowish-white flowers lined between each layer of red-coloured sepals. The flowers are usually removed and sliced very finely for use in Indian remedies and are purportedly effective for the purification of the urinary bladder and the treatment of urinary tract infection.

The banana fruit is also a great mood and energy booster, as it contains tryptophan, a type of protein that the body converts into serotonin — a chemical produced in the body and known to make one feel calm and relaxed. The high iron content in the banana fruit also stimulates the production of haemoglobins in the blood and are good for those suffering from anaemia. Snacking on bananas between meals helps to keep blood sugar levels up and reduce morning sickness for expectant ladies. In Ayurvedic medicine, bananas are prescribed for conditions such as gastric ulcers, gastritis and ulcerative colitis as they are gentle on the stomach.

Bananas are also rich in B vitamins which help calm the nervous system. Potassium is a vital mineral for normalising the heartbeat, sending oxygen to the brain and regulating the body's water content. When stressed, an individual's metabolic rate will usually increase, thereby reducing the potassium level in the body. The potassium level in the body can be restored to normal with a high-potassium banana snack. As the banana fruit is high in potassium yet low in sodium content, it is the perfect food for those suffering from high blood pressure. Even banana skins have healing properties; try rubbing insect bites with the inside of a banana skin to reduce swelling and provide relief.

Plantains are large, green bananas used for cooking. They contain more starch than regular bananas. Used in Indian medicine, plantains are good for providing energy and building tissue while removing heatiness at the same time. However, it is advised that those with a weak digestive system should not eat too many plantains as they are more difficult to digest.

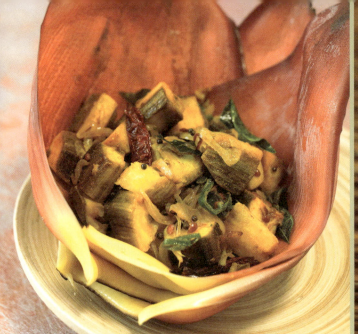
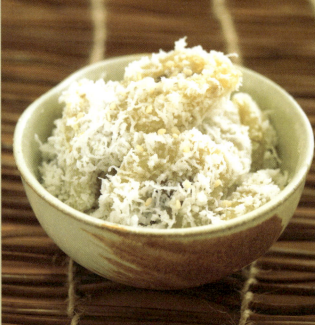

FROM LEFT TO RIGHT: Spicy Plantain (page 26), Steamed Bananas with Coconut (page 26) OPPOSITE: Banana Flowers with Yoghurt (page 27)

Spicy Plantain

Preparation time: 15 minutes
Cooking time: 15 minutes
Serves: 5

Plantains 5, medium, left unpeeled

Cooking oil 2 Tbsp

**Skinned split black lentils
    (urad** dhal) 1 tsp

Black mustard seeds 1 tsp

Dried chillies 3, cut into 2-cm
    (1-in) pieces

Onions 2, large, peeled and sliced

Green chillies 2, sliced

Curry leaves 2 sprigs, stems discarded

Turmeric powder 1 tsp

Cumin powder 1 tsp

Salt 1 1/2 tsp

Water 100 ml (3 1/3 fl oz / 3/8 cup)

Lime juice 1 Tbsp

**Chopped coriander (cilantro)
    leaves** 2 Tbsp

Boil enough water to cover plantains in a pot. Add plantains and boil for 10 minutes, then drain and leave to cool. Peel and cut into cubes.

Heat oil and fry lentils until golden brown. Add mustard seeds and dried chillies, then stir-fry until mustard seeds splutter.

Add onion slices, green chillies and curry leaves. Sauté until onions turn golden brown.

Stir in remaining ingredients and cook until all liquid is absorbed. Serve hot with rice, if desired.

Steamed Bananas with Coconut

Preparation time: 10 minutes
Steaming time: 20 minutes
Serves: 4

Bananas 4, large, left unpeeled

Freshly grated coconut 80 g (3 oz)

Fine salt 1/4 tsp

White sesame seeds 2 tsp,
    lightly toasted

Steam bananas over high heat for 20 minutes, then peel and cut into 1-cm (1/2-in) thick slices.

Mix grated coconut with salt and sesame seeds.

Sprinkle coconut mixture over steamed bananas and serve immediately. If preferred, roll banana slices in coconut mixture to coat well before serving as a dessert.

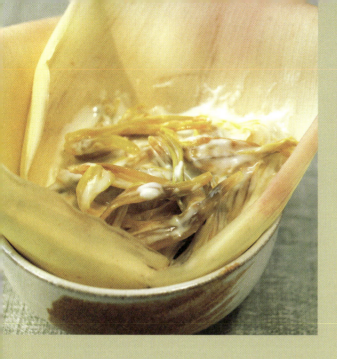

Banana Flowers with Yoghurt

This is considered an effective remedy for menstrual disorders. It seems that banana flowers increase progesterone which prevents excessive bleeding.

Banana flower bud 1, medium

Turmeric powder $^1/_2$ tsp

Low-fat yoghurt 200 ml (6 $^2/_3$ fl oz / $^3/_4$ cup)

Salt $^1/_4$ tsp

Ground black pepper $^1/_4$ tsp

Remove the red sepals and collect all the small flowers, discarding sepals. Chop flowers roughly.

Bring some water to the boil with turmeric powder. Boil chopped flowers for 5 minutes and drain well.

Combine boiled flowers with yoghurt, salt and pepper.

Remove and serve with other dishes. This remedy can be taken once daily.

Banana Appam

Preparation time: 15 minutes
Cooking time: 15 minutes
Serves: 6

Chopped jaggery 170 g (6 oz)

Water 250 ml (8 fl oz / 1 cup)

Rice flour 500 g (1 lb 1$^1/_2$ oz)

Salt $^1/_2$ tsp

Melted ghee (clarified butter) 2 tsp

Cardamom powder $^1/_2$ tsp

Finely chopped coconut chips 100 g (3$^1/_2$ oz)

Ripe bananas 6, large, peeled and coarsely mashed

Thick coconut milk 150 ml (5 fl oz / $^5/_8$ cup) (see page 50)

Oil or ghee (clarified butter) for greasing pan

Boil jaggery and water until jaggery dissolves. Strain and cool syrup.

Place syrup and remaining ingredients except oil into a large mixing bowl. Combine well to form a batter of dropping consistency.

Grease and heat a flat–based frying pan. Pour in a ladleful of batter and swirl pan so batter is evenly spread out.

Cook until batter is set and lightly browned on the underside, then turn over to brown the other side. Remove cooked pancake and repeat until batter is used up. Serve hot as a dessert or light snack.

Beetroot

The red beetroot, appreciated for its vibrant red colour which serves as a natural food colouring, is widely used in Indian cooking. Indeed, modern-day research has indicated that brightly-hued vegetables such as beetroots are rich in antioxidants and flavonoids that repair body cells and tissue, and reduce one's susceptibility to illnesses such as heart disease and cancer.

The beetroot is a rich source of natural sugars, carbohydrate, sodium, potassium, folic acid, iron and other trace minerals. When boiling beetroot, it is advisable to leave the skin on to prevent the colour from leaching into the water. Beetroot leaves have antibacterial properties. To treat inflammation of the skin and pimples, simply boil the leaves in water, leave to cool and then dab the affected areas with it to provide relief.

The iron-rich beetroot is regarded as an excellent blood tonic for the treatment of anaemia. It is also believed in Ayurvedic healing that beetroots are 'warming' for the body and thus make good food for cold climates. For those who suffer from chronic constipation, a daily drink of beetroot juice is recommended as it increases peristalsis which aids in purging waste from the system.

Common Beetroot
Sanskrit Chukunda
Tamil Kilangu
Botanical Beta vulgaris

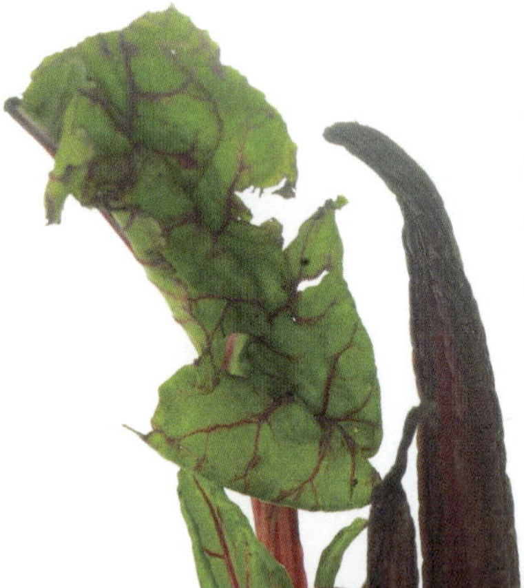

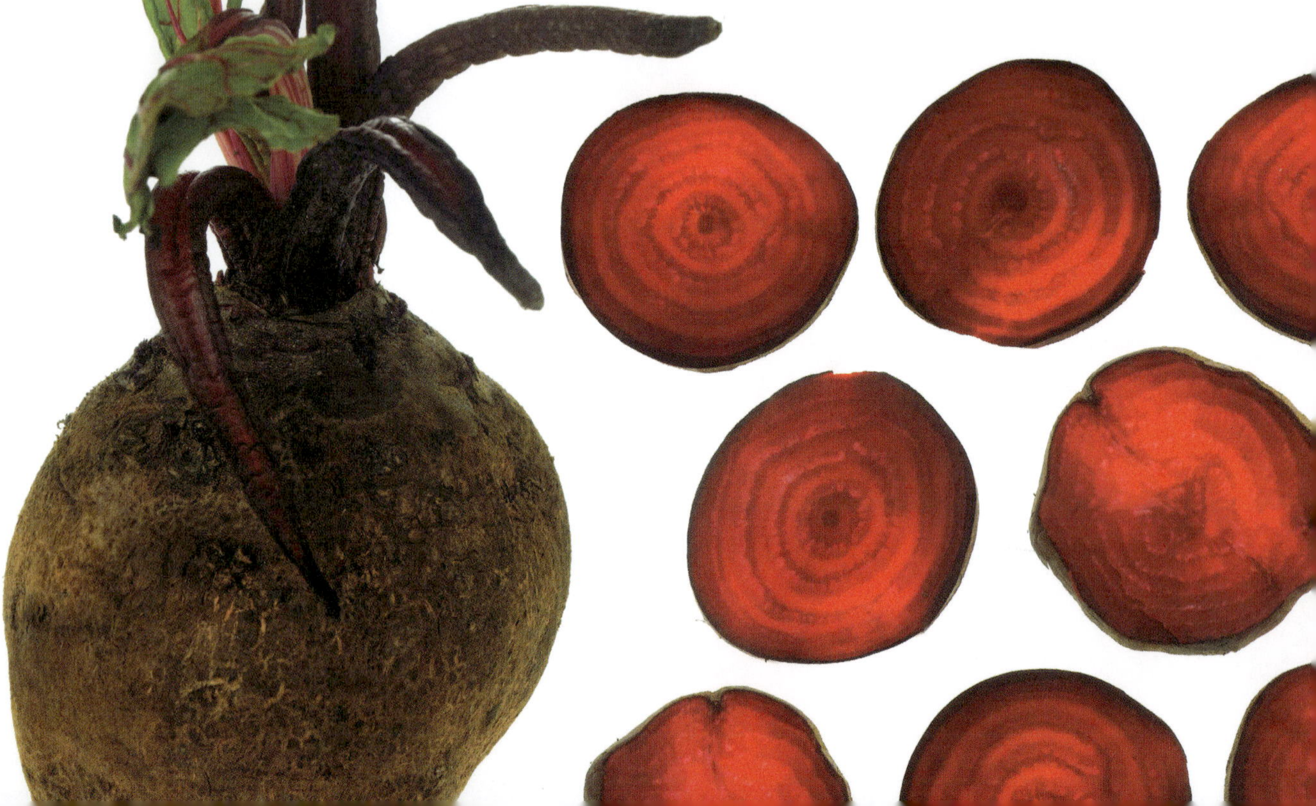

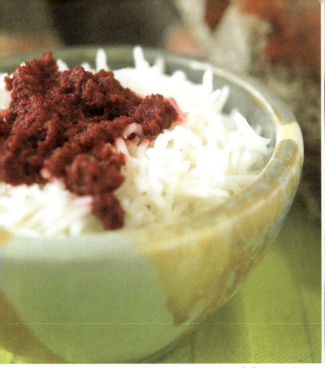
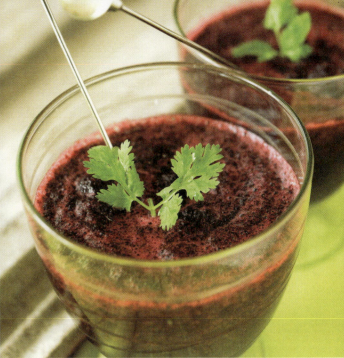

FROM LEFT TO RIGHT: *Beetroot Chutney (page 29), Remedy for Anaemia (page 29)*

Beetroot Chutney

Preparation time: 15 minutes
Cooking time: 5 minutes
Serves: 6

**Cooking oil or ghee
(clarified butter)** 1 Tbsp

**Split dried chickpeas
(*channa* dhal)** 1 tsp

**Skinned split black lentils
(*urad* dhal)** 1 tsp

Beetroot 350 g (12$^1/_2$ oz), peeled
and coarsely grated

Red chillies 4, cut into 2-cm
(1-in) pieces

Curry leaves 1 sprig, stem discarded

Tamarind pulp 50 g (2 oz), mixed with
200 ml (6$^2/_3$ fl oz / $^3/_4$ cup) water
and strained

Salt 1$^1/_4$ tsp

Heat oil and fry chickpeas and lentils until golden brown.

Add grated beetroot, chillies and curry leaves, then sauté for 4 minutes. Remove from heat and leave to cool slightly.

Blend (process) beetroot mixture with tamarind juice and salt to obtain a coarse paste. Serve with rice, chapati or bread.

Remedy for Anaemia

Drinking this daily helps to stimulate the production of red blood cells and reduce fatigue.

Beetroot 150 g (5$^1/_2$ oz) peeled
and cubed

**Chopped coriander (cilantro)
leaves** 2 Tbsp

Water 250 ml (8 fl oz / 1 cup)

Salt a pinch

Blend (process) all ingredients until smooth and drink immediately.

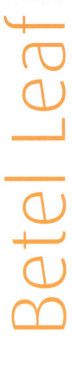

Betel Leaf

Common: Betel leaves, Pan leaves
Sanskrit: Tambula
Tamil: Paan
Botanical name: Piper betle

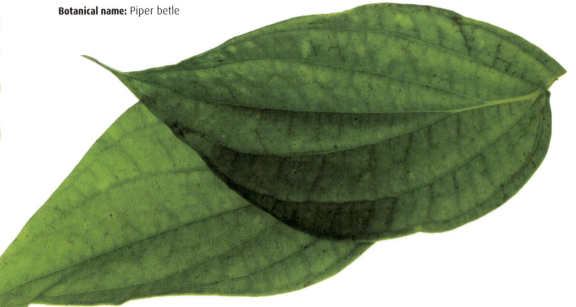

The shiny, heart-shaped leaves of the slender aromatic betel plant, are chewed by the older generation of Indians with an assortment of spices. It is a practice that is believed to strengthen the teeth and gums as well as provide relief for coughs and asthma. To make a betel-leaf chew, the leaf is smeared with lime paste and topped with spices that include betel nuts, saffron strands, cardamom, nutmeg, cloves and fennel. The leaf is then rolled up into a neat package called 'Paan' or 'Bida' and chewed.

With a content that includes calcium, carotene and vitamin C, the leaves have many traditional healing applications and are used for the relief of conditions such as headaches, arthritis and joint pain, where the leaves are simply applied directly onto the affected areas. The leaves can be used to brew a tea that helps keep the body odour-free when drunk. As betel leaves have strong antiseptic properties, they are crushed and applied to cuts and wounds, or made into poultices to treat boils. Many Indian home remedies for improving digestion and relieving flatulence use betel leaves.

Mouth Gargle

For a fresh, clean breath, gargle with the following natural remedy.

Betel leaves 10, coarsely chopped

Water 500 ml (16 fl oz / 2 cups)

Boil leaves in water for 5 minutes and set aside to cool.

When cool, strain mixture and gargle with liquid.

Remedy for Urinary Tract Infection

Take this remedy to alleviate a burning sensation when urinating.

Betel leaves 6

Milk 250 ml (8 fl oz / 1 cup)

Honey 1 Tbsp

Using mortar and pestle, pound betel leaves.

Wrap pounded leaves in a piece of muslin cloth and squeeze to extract juice.

Stir in milk and honey. Drink this portion twice daily until symptoms clear.

Tea to Aid Digestion

Betel leaves 8

Black peppercorns $^1/_2$ tsp, lightly crushed

Water 500 ml (16 fl oz /2 cups)

Boil all ingredients together in a pot for 10 minutes.

Strain mixture and drink 250 ml (8 fl oz /1 cup) tea each time, twice daily.

Elderly people who suffer from rheumatic pain in the knees may want to try this remedy. Warm some mustard oil and spread a thin layer on a few betel leaves. Place the leaves, oiled side on the knees, until the pain subsides. For the relief of headaches, grind the betel leaves into a pulp and apply on the temples. Leave on until headache subsides. A poultice of betel leaves can also be applied to relieve skin rash caused by an allergic reaction to certain cosmetics.

FROM LEFT TO RIGHT: Remedy for Urinary Tract Infection (page 31), Tea to Aid Digestion (page 31)

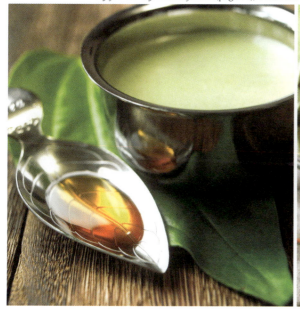
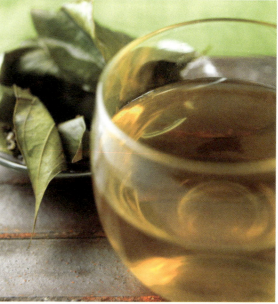

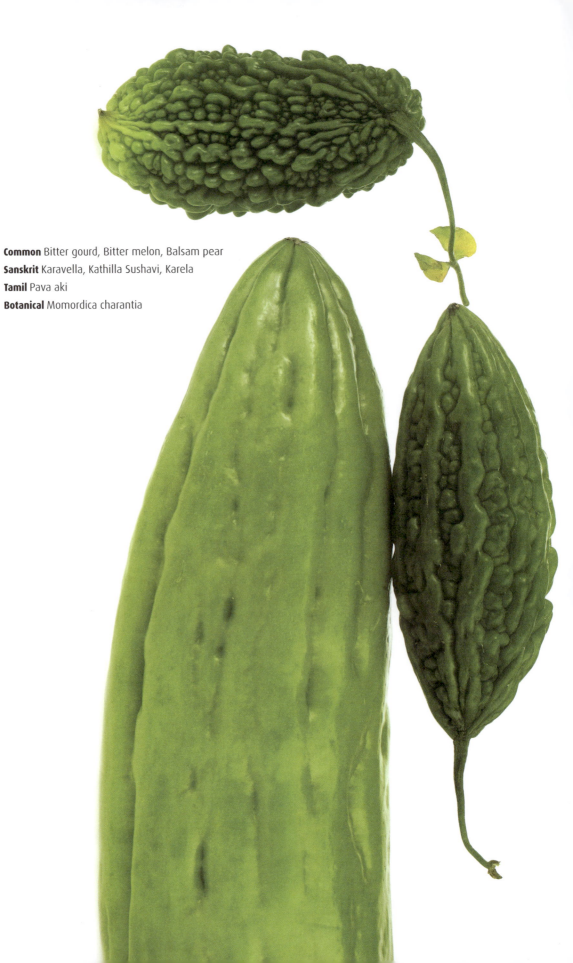

Bitter Gourd

Common Bitter gourd, Bitter melon, Balsam pear
Sanskrit Karavella, Kathilla Sushavi, Karela
Tamil Pava aki
Botanical Momordica charantia

A long, wrinkly-looking melon, the bitter gourd is ridged and tapered at both ends. It is cultivated in many countries, including China, India and Africa, with short, medium and long varieties available. The physical characteristics of the vegetable range from long, oblong and pale green to small, ovalish and dark green in colour. There is also a white variety available commercially. As its name suggests, the bitter gourd is a bitter-tasting vegetable and thus an acquired taste for many people.

Regarded as a treasury of medicinal virtues in Indian healing traditions, the bitter gourd is known to help regulate one's blood sugar level and is therefore beneficial for the diabetic. The melon is also purported to stimulate appetite and improve digestion. Rich in vitamins A, B, C and iron, the bitter gourd also aids in the treatment of medical conditions such as hypertension and neuritis as well as the build-up of the body's resistance against infection when eaten regularly.

To prepare a bitter gourd for cooking, wash it thoroughly, then halve lengthways, scrape out the seeds from the core and discard the seeds. Slice the vegetable according to the requirements of the recipe. To reduce the bitterness of the melon, blanch for three to four minutes in boiling water to which a few pinches of salt have been added. Drain and use as required.

Many Indian folk remedies prescribing the use of bitter gourds are available. It is believed that a daily drink of bitter gourd juice mixed with water helps to get rid of intestinal worms. To relieve piles, a daily dosage of three teaspoons of the juice of bitter gourd leaves mixed with one glass of buttermilk, is prescribed to be taken for a month until symptoms subside. Drinking the juice extracted from pounded bitter gourd leaves is also believed to treat alcoholism.

Possessing antibacterial properties, the bitter gourd has a beneficial effect in the treatment of scabies, psoriasis, ringworms and other fungal diseases. A common remedy for these conditions is one cupful of fresh bitter gourd juice mixed with a teaspoonful of lime juice, to be sipped on an empty stomach daily for up to six months.

The roots of the bitter gourd plant have been a folk medicine for respiratory disorders since ancient times. One remedy calls for a teaspoonful of the paste of the roots to be mixed with an equal amount of honey or basil leaf juice and taken for up to a month daily to treat asthma, bronchitis, pharyngitis and colds. A paste of the roots of the bitter gourd plant can also be applied over external piles to bring relief.

Stir-fried Bitter Gourd

Preparation time: 30 minutes
Cooking time: 10 minutes
Serves: 5

Bitter gourd 800 g (1³/₄ lb), halved lengthways, pith removed and thinly sliced across

Salt 1¹/₂ tsp

Turmeric powder 1¹/₂ tsp

Cooking oil for deep-frying

Skinned split black lentils (urad dhal) 1 tsp

Black mustard seeds 1 tsp

Onion 1, large, peeled and finely chopped

Curry leaves 2 sprigs, stems discarded

Chilli powder 1 tsp

Coriander powder 1 tsp

Rub bitter gourd with salt and turmeric all over and set aside for 20 minutes.

Deep-fry bitter gourd in hot oil until golden brown and crispy. Drain on absorbent paper towels.

Leave 1¹/₂ Tbsp oil in the pan and stir-fry lentils until golden brown. Add mustard seeds and stir-fry until they stop spluttering.

Add onion and curry leaves then sauté until onion turns golden brown.

Stir in chilli and coriander powders and remove from heat immediately. Add fried bitter gourd and stir to mix well. Serve hot with rice and other dishes.

Jaundice Remedy

Bitter gourd 60 g (2 oz), seeded

Water 60 ml (2 fl oz / ¹/₄ cup)

Lemon juice 1 tsp

Blend all ingredients in a blender (processor) until smooth.

Strain if desired and drink immediately. Take this remedy once daily until the yellow tinge in the eyes subsides.

Stuffed Bitter Gourd

Preparation time: 1 hour
Cooking time: 15 minutes
Serves: 5

Bitter gourd 5, small, left whole

Chickpea flour (besan) 1¹/₂ Tbsp

Onions 2, medium, peeled and coarsely chopped

Garlic 6 cloves, peeled and coarsely chopped

Green chillies 4, coarsely chopped

Ginger 3-cm (1¹/₂-in) knob, peeled and coarsely chopped

Roasted cumin powder 1¹/₂ Tbsp

Coriander powder 1¹/₂ Tbsp

Turmeric powder 1 tsp

Grated skinned, unripe mango 100 g (3 ¹/₂ oz)

Sugar 1 tsp

Salt 1 tsp

Cooking oil for frying

Boil enough water in pot to cover bitter gourd and add a pinch of salt. Add bitter gourd and boil until slightly soft. Drain and set aside to cool.

Slit each bitter gourd lengthways and discard seeds.

Rub 1 tsp chickpea flour all over the inside and outside of each bitter gourd. Set aside for 20 minutes.

Put onions, garlic, chillies and ginger into a large bowl. Stir in remaining ingredients except bitter gourd and oil. Mix well.

Stuff each bitter gourd with onion mixture tightly. To prevent mixture from falling out, secure both ends of each bitter gourd with kitchen string.

Deep-fry stuffed bitter gourd in hot oil until golden brown. Discard kitchen string and serve immediately with rice and other dishes.

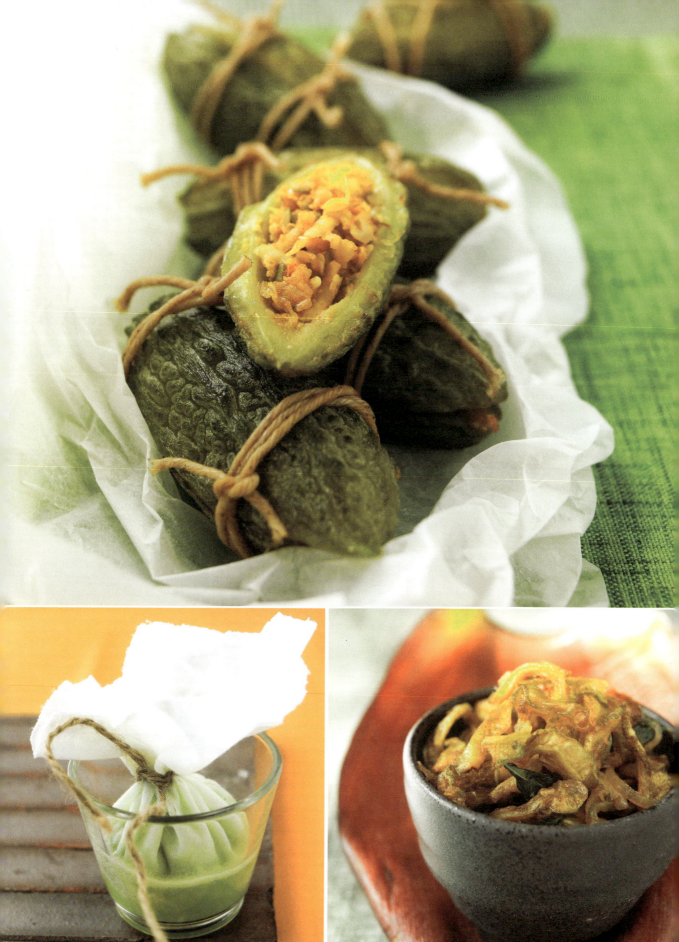

Black Mustard Seed

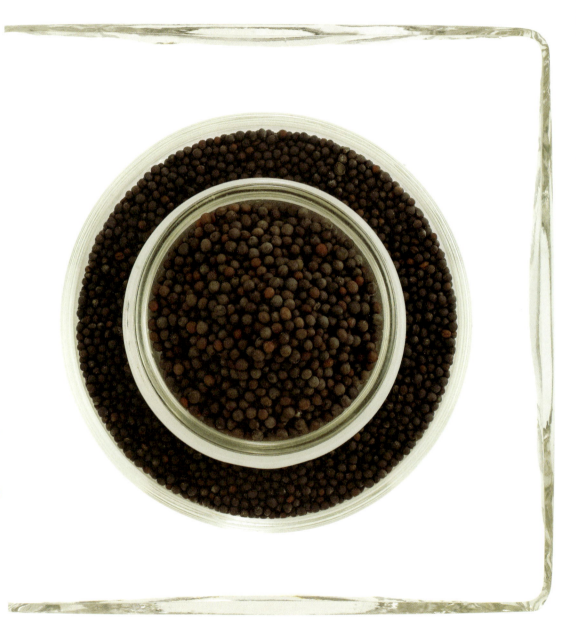

Common Black mustard seeds
Sanskrit Krishnika, Krishnasarshapa
Tamil Kadugu
Botanical Brassica nigra

Although mustard seeds are available in black, brown and white varieties, black mustard seeds are more important as a spice in India. Both the seeds as well as the oil pressed from the seeds are commonly used in Indian recipes and remedies.

The hot-tasting flavour and pungency of the spice is released in the form of an essential oil when the crushed seeds are mixed with water. To extract the nutty fragrance of black mustard seeds, simply fry them in a little hot oil until they splutter before adding to dishes such as pickles and curries.

Black mustard seeds are one of the oldest spices to be used in Indian folk medicine. In the villages, mustard poultices are commonly used as an antidote for scorpion stings. Hot mustard plasters are used to treat respiratory conditions such as chest pains, coughs and shortness of breath. The pungent and bitter spice is known to promote digestion by stimulating the secretion of gastric juices when used in small quantities as a condiment. It also helps lower high blood pressure.

To treat arthritis, warm some mustard oil and smear over some betel leaves before placing the leaves, with the oiled side on the affected joints. Wrap a clean cotton bandage over the leaves and joint for a few hours to provide relief. Mustard powder is also added to warm water to make a therapeutic footbath for soothing tired feet.

As mustard seeds contain emetic properties which induces vomiting, drinking a teaspoonful of crushed mustard seeds mixed in a glass of water will help to purge poison or drugs from a person's system within 10 minutes.

Mustard Oil Hair Conditioner

This remedy is helpful in encouraging the growth of abundant hair.

Mustard oil 500 ml (16 fl oz / 2 cups)

Henna leaves 100 g (3¹/₂ oz)
  or henna powder 2 Tbsp

Boil all ingredients together for about 15 minutes.

Cool thoroughly and filter through a piece of clean muslin cloth. Store in a sterilised glass bottle in a dark place.

Apply 1 Tbsp oil onto scalp and massage into hair.

Leave on for 1 hour, then rinse and shampoo as per usual.

Note: For best effect, use this treatment twice a week. The oil can be kept for up to 1 year.

Remedy for Scabies

Mustard oil 250 ml (8 fl oz / 1 cup)

Crushed dried neem leaves 1 Tbsp

Turmeric powder 2 tsp

Mix all ingredients together and apply all over the body. Leave on for about 1 hour, then rinse off and shower as per usual.

Chilli Mustard Pickle

Preparation time: 15 minutes
Cooking time: 4 minutes
Serves: 10

Mustard oil 200 ml
(6²/₃ fl oz / ³/₄ cup)

Black mustard seeds 70 g (2¹/₂ oz), coarsely pounded

Asafoetida powder 1¹/₂ tsp

Turmeric powder 2 tsp

Powdered black salt 25 g (1 oz)

Large green chillies 300 g (10¹/₂ oz), cut into 1-cm (¹/₂-in) pieces

Rice vinegar 200 ml (6²/₃ fl oz / ³/₄ cup)

Sugar 1 Tbsp

Heat oil in a large stainless steel pan. Remove from heat. Add all remaining ingredients and combine well.

Allow to cool thoroughly and store in sterilised, airtight glass jars. Serve with other dishes after 3 days.

Note: This pickle can be kept refrigerated for up to 6 months.

Vermicelli Uppuma

Preparation time: 20 minutes
Cooking time: 15 minutes
Serves: 6

Ghee (clarified butter) 2 tsp + 1 Tbsp

Indian wheat-flour vermicelli 500 g (1 lb 1¹/₂ oz)

Cooking oil 1 Tbsp

Skinned split black lentils (*urad* dhal) 1 tsp

Split dried chickpeas (*channa* dhal) 1 Tbsp

Cashew nuts 120g (4¹/₂ oz), chopped

Black mustard seeds 1¹/₂ tsp

Dried chillies 3, cut into 2-cm (1-in) pieces

Onion 1, peeled and chopped

Ginger 2-cm (1-in) knob, peeled and finely minced

Green chillies 2, cut into 2-cm (1-in) pieces

Curry leaves 2 sprigs, stems discarded

Asafoetida powder 1 tsp

Water 900 ml (28¹/₂ fl oz / 3⁵/₈ cups)

Natural yoghurt 100 ml
(3¹/₃ fl oz / ³/₈ cup)

Salt 2 tsp

Mixed vegetables 300 g (10¹/₂ oz)

Lime juice 2 Tbsp

Heat 2 tsp ghee and stir-fry vermicelli for a minute until it turns a shade darker. Set aside.

In a separate large pan, heat oil together with 1 Tbsp ghee and fry lentils, chickpeas and cashew nuts until golden brown.

Add mustard seeds and dried chillies, and fry until mustard seeds stop spluttering. Add onion, ginger, chillies, curry leaves and asafoetida powder. Sauté for 1 minute or until aromatic. Stir in water, yoghurt, salt and mixed vegetables. Bring to the boil for 2 minutes.

Add vermicelli to pan, combine well and cook over medium heat until all liquid has been absorbed and vermicelli is cooked. Sprinkle lime juice all over, stir to combine well and dish out. Serve hot as a light meal or with other dishes.

CLOCKWISE FROM TOP: Vermicelli Uppuma (page 38) , Mustard Oil Hair Conditioner (page 37), Chilli Mustard Pickle (page 38)

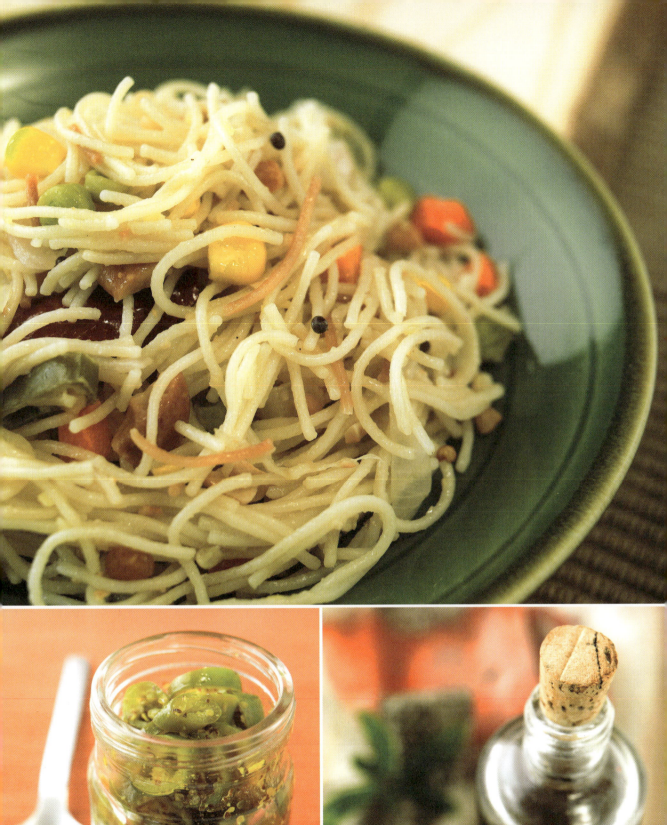
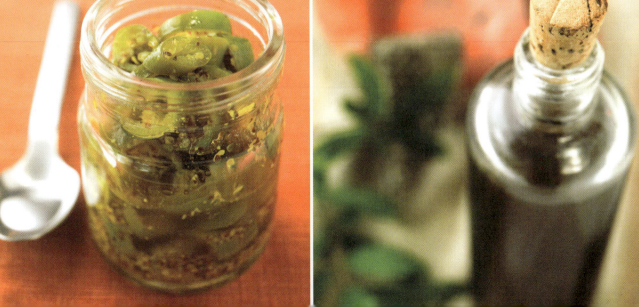

Cabbage

One of the most highly-rated leafy vegetables available, the cabbage is a rich source of nutrients including vitamin C, potassium, folic acid and antioxidants. In India, white cabbages are widely used and are delicious, whether served raw in salads or quickly stir-fried to retain a tender yet slightly crisp texture. Avoid slicing cabbages in advance as the vitamin C content of the vegetable will dissipate rapidly. If slicing the vegetable way before cooking is a must, store in a plastic bag, then seal tightly and refrigerate until ready to use.

Common Cabbage
Sanskrit Patta gobhi
Tamil Muttai kos
Botanical Brassica oleracea

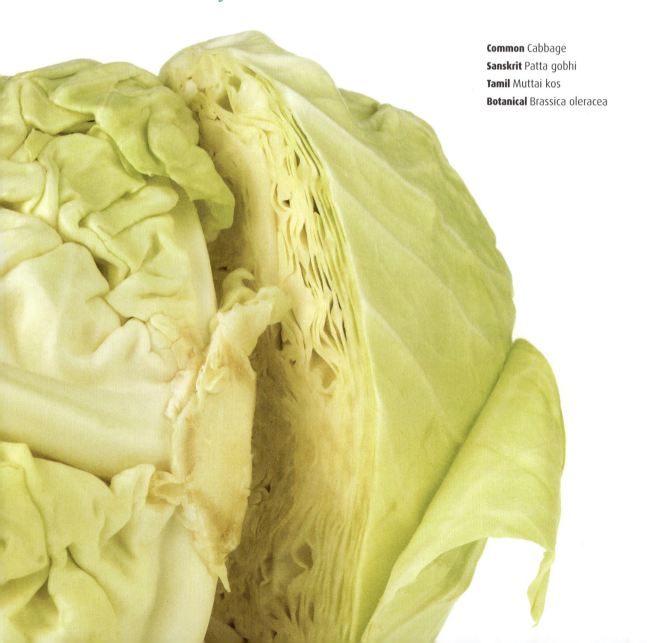

In traditional Indian medicine, the cabbage is considered useful in regulating the blood sugar level and treating disorders of the urinary system as well as some skin diseases. Cabbages are also regarded as beneficial for the stomach; some Indians drink cabbage juice neat to cleanse the mucous membranes of the stomach and the gastro-intestinal tract. As cabbages are high in fibre, a cabbage salad is an excellent cure for constipation.

In the arena of external medicinal applications, many Indians use cabbage leaves as compresses for the treatment of ulcers, sores, blisters, psoriasis and minor burns. To prepare a compress, choose the thickest and greenest outer leaves of the cabbage as they have the most effective healing property. Use the leaves whole. They should be washed thoroughly in warm water and dried with a clean towel. If the leaves are very stiff, make them more pliable by removing the thick veins and running a rolling pin over the leaves. Place the leaves, with the inside layers on the affected body part in an overlapping manner. Hold the leaves in place by wrapping a clean piece of cotton or lint-free cloth around the affected part. Finally, secure the entire compress firmly by covering with cling film or an elastic bandage. The compress can be kept on for the whole day and overnight. If the leaves wilt or change colour, simply discard and replace with fresh leaves. When changing to a fresh compress, the affected area should be thoroughly washed and dried before the application.

For lactating mothers who suffer from engorgement, cabbage leaves can also be applied as a compress to relieve the condition. Prepare a cabbage compress as described and refrigerate for up to half an hour before use. To hold the cabbage leaves in place, tuck the leaves into the bra to cover the breasts, leaving the nipples exposed. Leave on for two hours or until the cabbage leaves wilt. Replace with fresh cabbage leaves if necessary.

Cabbage Tuvayal

Preparation time: 15 minutes
Cooking time: 5 minutes
Serves: 6

Cooking oil 1½ Tbsp

Coriander seeds 2 Tbsp

Green chillies 5, cut into 2-cm (1-in) pieces

Cumin seeds 2 tsp

Curry leaves 3 sprigs, stems discarded

Cabbage 500 g (1 lb 1½ oz), finely shredded

Tamarind pulp 80 g (3 oz), mixed with 80 ml (2½ fl oz / ⅓ cup) water and strained

Salt 1½ tsp

Heat oil and fry coriander seeds and green chillies until aromatic.

Add cumin seeds, curry leaves, cabbage, tamarind juice and salt. Sauté for 5 minutes.

Cool thoroughly and blend (process) mixture in a blender (processor) to obtain a coarse texture. Serve with rice and other dishes.

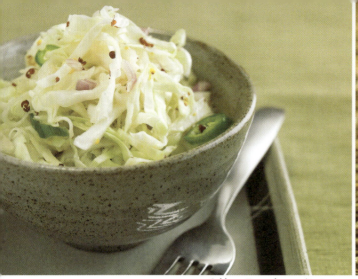
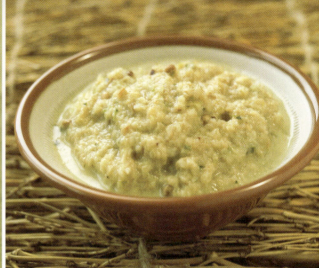

FROM LEFT TO RIGHT: Cabbage Tuvayal (page 41), Lazeez Bandh (page 42) OPPOSITE: *Stir-fried Cabbage (page 42)*

Lazeez Bandh (Cabbage Salad)

Preparation time: 15 minutes
Cooking time: 2 minutes
Serves: 4

Cabbage 350 g (12^1/$_2$ oz), very finely chopped

Green chillies 2, sliced

Onion 1, medium, peeled and finely chopped

Salad Dressing

Water 50 ml (1^2/$_3$ fl oz / ^{1}/$_4$ cup)

White vinegar 4 Tbsp

Salt 2 tsp

Sugar 2 Tbsp

Black mustard seeds 2 tsp, coarsely pounded

Prepare salad dressing. Put water, vinegar, salt, sugar and mustard seeds into a pot and bring to the boil for 1 minute.

Remove from heat and cool to lukewarm.

Put cabbage, green chillies and onion into a salad bowl and pour prepared dressing over.

Toss well and chill for at least 1 hour before serving as a light appetiser.

Stir-fried Cabbage

Preparation time: 15 minutes
Cooking time: 15 minutes
Serves: 4

Cooking oil 2 Tbsp

Skinned split black lentils (*urad* dhal) 1 tsp

Black mustard seeds 1 tsp

Onion 1, medium, peeled and finely chopped

Green chillies 2, stalks discarded and left whole

Dried red chillies 2, left whole

Curry leaves 2 sprigs, stems discarded

Cabbage 750 g (1 lb 10 oz), finely shredded

Turmeric powder 1 tsp

Salt 1^1/$_4$ tsp

Freshly grated coconut 50 g (2 oz)

Heat oil in a pan and fry lentils until golden brown and aromatic. Add mustard seeds and fry until they splutter.

Add onion, chillies and curry leaves, then sauté until onion turns golden brown.

Add cabbage, turmeric powder and salt. Cook, covered, stirring occasionally until cabbage is cooked.

Stir in coconut and remove from heat. Serve hot with rice.

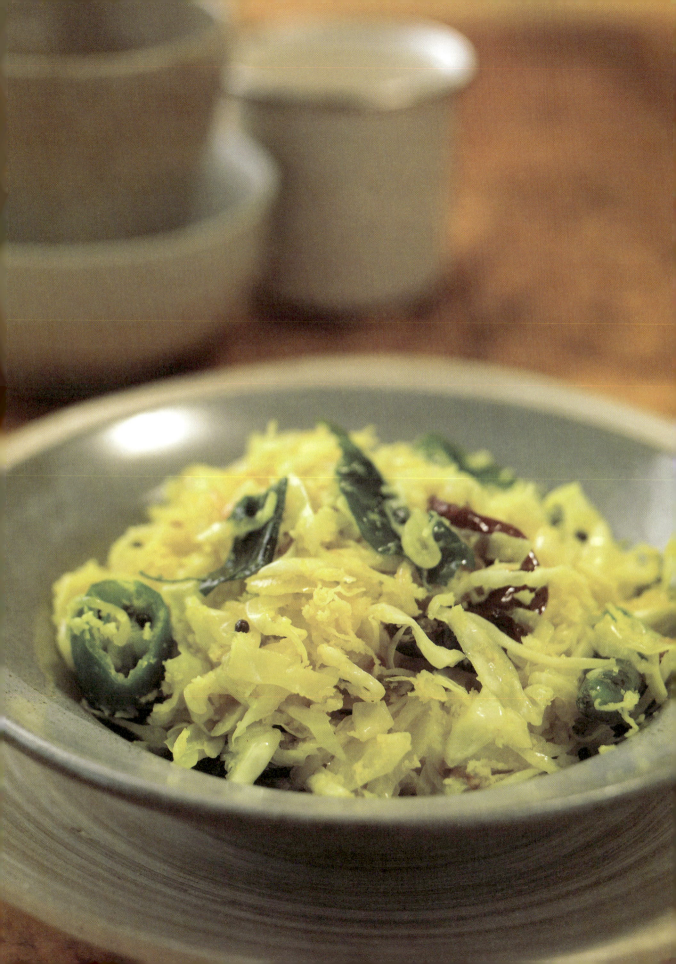

Cardamom

Common Cardamom
Sanskrit Ela, Ellka, Suksmaila
Tamil Aila cheddi, Elakkai, Yelakkai
Botanical Eletteria cardamomum

Cardamoms are derived from a ginger-like plant. They are available in two varieties: large brownish-black pods and small green pods. Bleached white pods are also commercially available and are of the cheaper variety as the bleaching process has partly removed the efficacy of the spice.

Each pod contains three double rows of brownish-black sticky seeds. The pod is almost oval-shaped and has the texture of thick, tough paper. The surface of the cardamom pod is rough; the brownish-black cardamom has a wrinkly skin.

Cardamoms are available whole or ground into powder. It is better to buy whole pods rather than powder as the latter loscs its flavour very quickly. Considered the queen of spices, the cardamom has a warm, pungent smell that is a cross between the aromas of camphor and eucalyptus, and leaves a warm, bittersweet taste in the mouth when consumed.

In India, cardamoms are used for flavouring curries, cakes, breads and other culinary delights such as coffee and confectionery. The cardamom is also the classic spice that makes the masala tea world-famous. To fully release the flavour of the seeds, they should be dry-roasted before use. Simply split open the pods, remove the seeds and discard the pods. Heat a clean and dry pan and dry-roast the seeds until fragrant. The seeds can then be lightly pounded before they are added to the main ingredients when cooking, or ground with other spices as required. Keep the pods whole until ready to use, to retain maximum flavour. If using whole pods, remove immediately after cooking as they can leave an unpleasant bitter taste when left in the dish for too long.

The aromatic and therapeutic properties of the cardamom are attributed to its volatile oil content. Traditional home remedies made with cardamoms include preparations for relieving flatulence, aiding digestion and soothing coughs.

Cough Buster

Holy basil leaves 10 g ($^1/_3$ oz)
Long pepper 10 g ($^1/_3$ oz)
Cardamoms 20 g ($^2/_3$ oz)
Honey $^1/_2$ tsp

Grind all ingredients except honey together into a fine powder.

Mix $^1/_2$ tsp ground mixture with $^1/_2$ tsp honey. Consume this portion thrice a day until coughing stops.

FROM LEFT TO RIGHT: *Cough Buster (page 45), Cardamom Tea (page 46)*

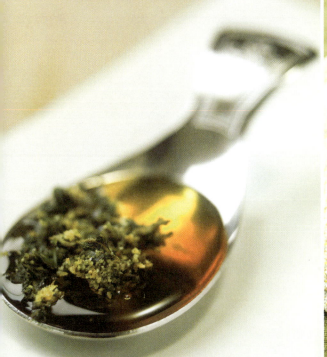
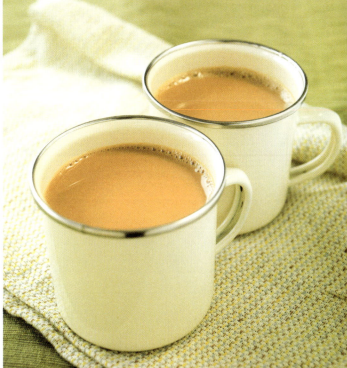

Cardamom Tea

Cardamom is reputed to increase appetite and soothe the mucous membrane. This tea helps to relieve gas and heartburn and also aids digestion.

Preparation time: 5 minutes
Cooking time: 2 minutes
Serves: 8

Dried tea leaves 1 Tbsp

Cardamoms 10, pounded

Water 1.25 l (40 fl oz / 5 cups)

Sugar to taste

Hot milk to taste

Place tea leaves, cardamoms and water in a pot and bring to the boil for 2 minutes.

Strain tea and serve with sugar and milk on the side as desired.

Cardamom Flavoured Puffed Rice

Preparation time: 10 minutes
Cooking time: 20 minutes
Serves: 4

Jaggery 300 g (10^1/$_2$ oz), grated

Water 100 ml (3^1/$_2$ fl oz / ^{3}/$_8$ cup)

Puffed rice 550 g (1 lb 3^1/$_2$ oz)

Roasted skinned split black lentils (*urad* dhal) 30 g (1 oz)

Roasted peanuts 40 g (1^1/$_2$ oz)

Roasted cashew nuts 40 g (1^1/$_2$ oz), crushed

Cardamoms 10, pounded

Put jaggery and water into a pan and boil until syrup becomes thick and reaches temperature of about 115°C (240°F), with soft-ball consistency.

Put the rest of the ingredients into a mixing bowl. Pour syrup little by little over mixture, mixing constantly and quickly until well-coated with syrup.

Transfer mixture onto a baking tray, flatten quickly with the back of a spoon and leave to cool and set before breaking into serving-sized pieces. Store in an airtight container. Serve as a snack.

Note: To test consistency of syrup: pour a little syrup onto a plate. The consistency is right if you can pick it up and roll the thickened syrup into a ball.

Sore Throat Gargle

As cardamoms are breath fresheners, some Indian restaurants serve cardamoms and fennel seeds after a meal for customers to chew on and freshen their breath. Gargle with this infusion of cardamoms to bring relief to sore throats.

Cardamoms 2 Tbsp

Water 1 litre (32 fl oz / 4 cups)

Salt 2 tsp

Pound cardamoms lightly to open up the pods and release the black seeds inside.

Place pounded cardamoms, water and salt in a pan and bring to the boil over medium heat for 5 minutes.

Strain and leave to cool before using as a gargle.

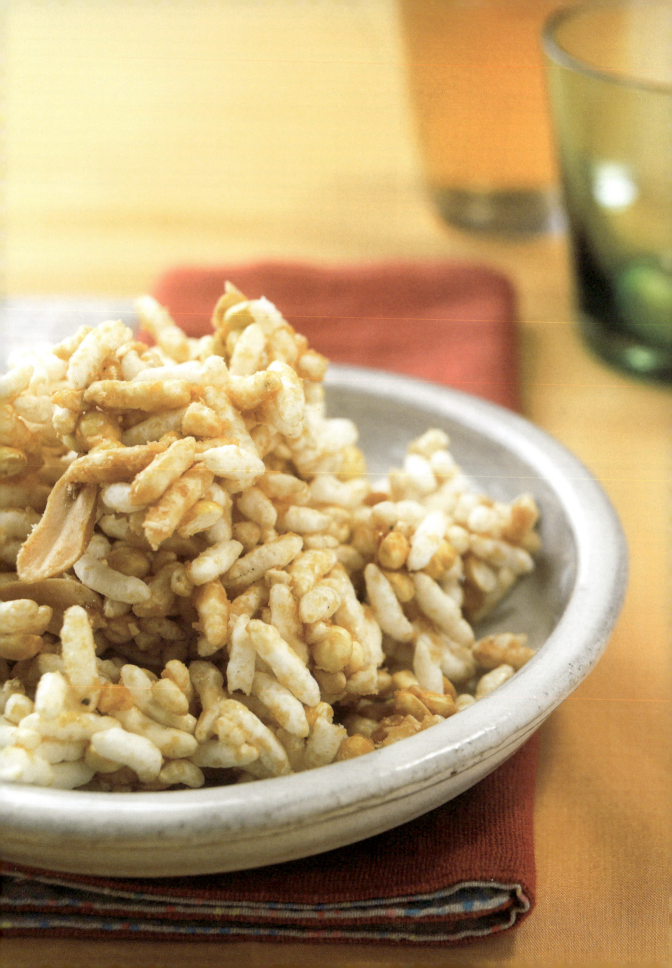

chilli

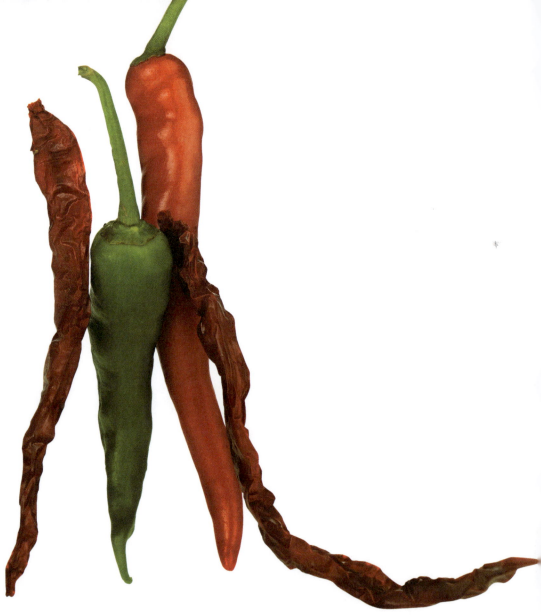

Common Chilli, Chilli pepper, Capsicum, Cayenne pepper, bird's-eye chilli
Sanskrit Katuvira, Marichiphala Ujjvala
Tamil Pachai milagai (green chillies), Sigappu milagai (red chillies)
Botanical Capsicum annuum var. annuum, Capsicum frutescens

An excellent source of vitamins A, B, C and E and minerals including folate, potassium and thiamin, chillies are available in many varieties, sizes, colours and degrees of pungency. In India, chillies are widely available as fresh and dried chillies, chili powder and pickled chillies. Scientific research has shown that eating chillies stimulates the release of endorphins which are natural painkillers, thus producing a calming effect in the body. This probably explains why chillies can be addictive for some people! To relieve the 'burning' sensation in the mouth upon eating chillies of high pungency, drink yoghurt or milk as the butterfat in these drinks will help dissolve the capsaicinoids (organic compounds responsible for the pungency of the chillies) from the lining of the mouth and tongue.

When using fresh chillies, remove the inside pithy white parts and seeds to reduce the pungency if desired, since capsaicinoids are found on these parts of the fruit. While the use of dried chillies in curries and seasonings is prevalent throughout India, fresh green chillies are more commonly used in South Indian cuisines.

In traditional Indian home remedies, chillies are often used to stimulate the appetite and aid digestion as they help detoxify the gastrointestinal tract. Chillies are also used to relieve nasal and lung congestion by increasing metabolism. It dilates the airway to reduce wheezing and breathing difficulties.

Hot Spiced Powder

Preparation time: 5 minutes
Cooking time: 5 minutes
Serves: 8

Gingelly oil 1 Tbsp

Split yellow lentils (*tur* dhal)
 50 g (2 oz)

Skinned split black lentils (*urad* dhal)
 120 g (4¹/₂ oz)

Curry leaves 5 sprigs, stems discarded

Dried chillies 25 g (1 oz)

Asafoetida powder 2 tsp

Garlic 5 cloves, peeled and sliced

Salt 2¹/₂ tsp

Heat oil and fry both types of dhal and curry leaves until dhal turns golden brown and curry leaves, crispy.

Add dried chillies towards the end to prevent them from getting burnt. Remove from heat and set aside to cool.

Grind dhal mixture with asafoetida powder in a coffee grinder without adding any water. Finally, add garlic and salt to mixture and grind to a coarse powder.

Place ground powder on absorbent paper towels to remove any trace of oil.

Store in an airtight container for up to 3 months. Use as a condiment for thosai, chapati or rice.

FROM LEFT TO RIGHT: *Chilli Chicken (page 50), Hot Spiced Powder (page 49)*

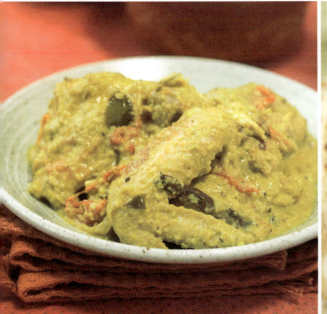
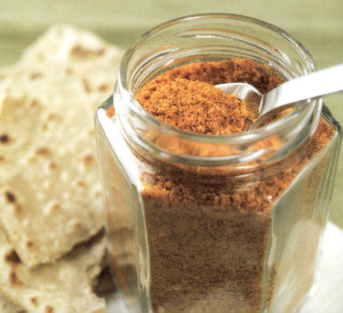

Chilli Chicken

Preparation time: 15 minutes
Cooking time: 15 minutes
Serves: 6

Chicken 1.5 kg (3 lb 4¹/₂ oz),
  skinned and cut into 15 pieces

Cooking oil 3 Tbsp

Cardamoms 5

Fennel seeds 1¹/₂ tsp,
  coarsely pounded

Onions 2, medium, peeled and sliced

Curry leaves 2 sprigs, stems discarded

Thick coconut milk 125 ml
  (4 fl oz / ¹/₂ cup) (see note)

Tomatoes 2, quartered

Salt 1 tsp

Marinade

Green chillies 10, finely chopped

Natural yoghurt 200 ml
  (6²/₃ fl oz / ³/₄ cup)

Ginger paste 2 Tbsp

Garlic paste 3 Tbsp

White peppercorns 2 tsp,
  coarsely ground

Meat curry powder 2 Tbsp

Salt 1 tsp

Place chicken and marinade ingredients into a large mixing bowl and combine well. Leave to marinate for 1 hour.

Heat oil and fry cardamoms and fennel seeds until aromatic.

Add onions and curry leaves and sauté until onions turn golden brown.

Add coconut milk, tomatoes, salt and chicken. Mix well and cook, stirring occasionally until sauce thickens and chicken is tender. Remove and serve hot with rice and other dishes.

Note: To make thick coconut milk, add 125 ml (4 fl oz / ¹/₂ cup) water to the freshly grated flesh of a coconut in a mixing bowl, then put mixture into a cheesecloth and squeeze firmly to extract all the liquid (yields about 750 ml–1 litre). To obtain thin coconut milk, place the squeezed coconut back into the bowl with 625 ml (20 fl oz / 2¹/₂ cups) water and repeat the process of squeezing through the cheesecloth to extract all the thin liquid. Use as required. For convenience, use packets of ready-to-use coconut milk of varying consistencies, which are now available at most Asian grocery stores.

Chilli Potato Poultice for Rheumatic Aches

As chillies stimulate the release of natural painkillers known as endorphins in the body, this remedy will help provide some relief of rheumatic pain.

Chilli powder 2 tsp

Potatoes 2, medium,
  cooked, peeled and mashed

Add chilli powder to mashed potatoes and mix well.

Wrap potato mixture in a piece of muslin cloth or cotton gauze to make a poultice.

Hold and lightly press poultice on affected body. If desired, flatten poultice slightly and wrap cling film (plastic wrap) around poultice and affected area to generate warmth. Remove after 1 hour.

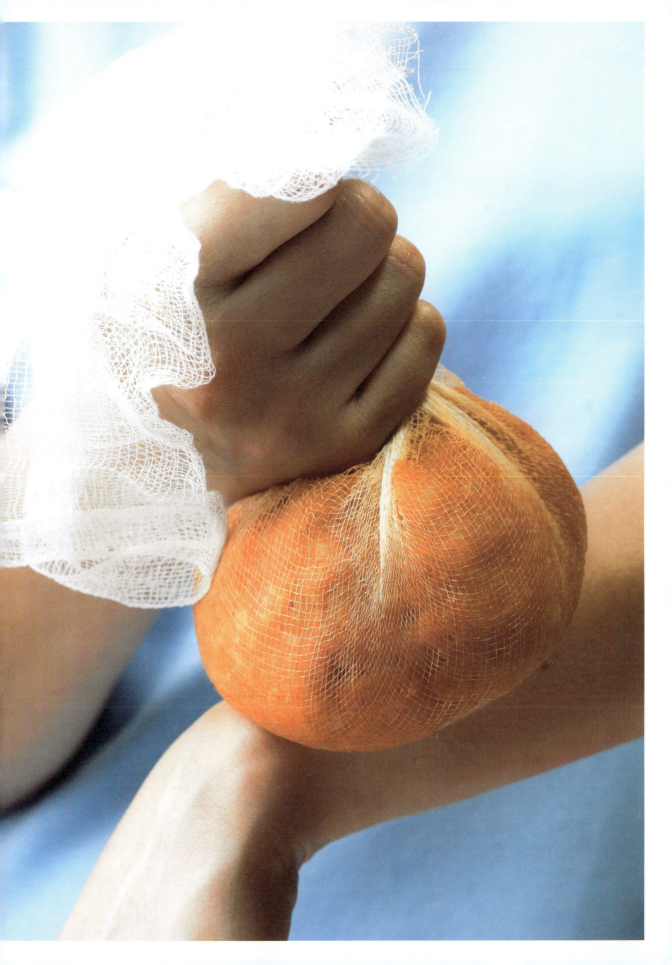

cinnamon

Common Ceylon cinnamon
Sanskrit Sthula, Taja, Tvak
Tamil Llavangam, Lavangapatri, Lavangapattai
Botanical Cinnamomum verum/ Cinnamomum zeylanicum
(native to Sri Lanka)

Common Chinese cinnamon / Cassia
Sanskrit Khasa, Khakasa
Tamil Gaehagesha kasakasa
Botanical Cinnamomum cassia/ Cinnamomum aromaticum
(cultivated mainly in China, limited cultivation in Tamil Nadu, wild in Mizoram)

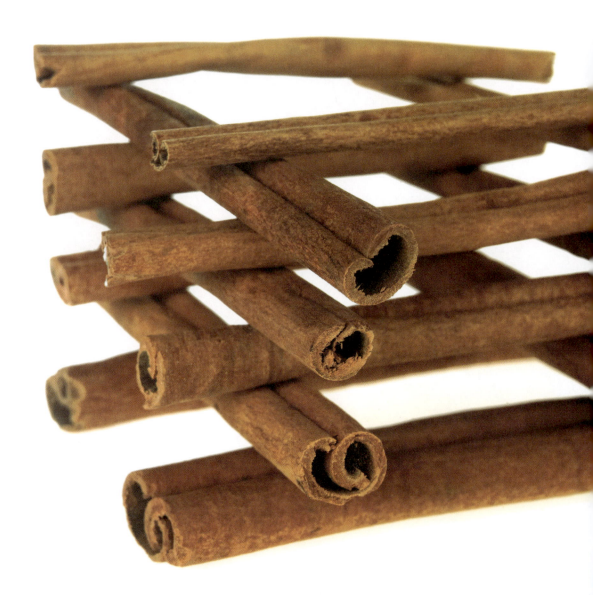

A highly aromatic spice, the cinnamon is the dried bark of evergreen trees and shrubs in the laurel family. One of the more common trees from which cinnamon is derived is the cassia or Chinese cinnamon tree; its bark is thick, rich in oil and dark brown in colour. Another variety, Ceylon cinnamon, is the thin, reddish-brown bark that is rich in oil and obtained from the tender branches of a shrub native to Sri Lanka.

While both types of cinnamon possess similar warm and sweet qualities, Chinese cinnamon or cassia, as it is commonly known, is more bitter and astringent in flavour, compared to Ceylon cinnamon, which has a more subtle and pleasant flavour. Given the more refined flavour of Ceylon cinnamon and the greater availability of the cassia, Ceylon cinnamon is hence more costly than cassia. Commercially available cinnamon powder is usually ground from the cheaper variety of cassia as well.

When buying cinnamon sticks, Ceylon cinnamon can be differentiated from cassia sticks from the way the bark is rolled. Ceylon cinnamon sticks are rolled in single quills whereas cassia sticks are rolled from both ends and resemble scrolls. While all types of cinnamon sticks have an indefinite shelf life, ground cinnamon should be kept refrigerated and used quickly as it is prone to losing its flavour. Despite the differences in their strength and quality, both types of cinnamon possess the same efficacy in their healing properties.

The aromatic spice is also used in a wide selection of Indian food including pickles, curries and confectioneries. A large number of Indian meat recipes also include the use of cinnamon as it is known for its preserving qualities. When cooking, fry cinnamon sticks in oil or ghee first to fully release the aromatic flavour of the spice in the dish.

In the home, the cinnamon has many useful applications. To make a natural freshener, mix a portion of ground cinnamon with an equal amount of bicarbonate of soda and sprinkle on the carpet before vacuuming. Storing a few cinnamon sticks with potatoes will also prevent them from sprouting.

As a medicinal spice, the main properties of cinnamon are astringent, carminative, and antiseptic. Remedies using cinnamon powder are often used for treating skin rashes and flatulence, while cinnamon oil, which is a natural anaesthetic, is used in tiny quantities for relieving toothaches. To treat small cuts, wash and pat dry then sprinkle a little ground cinnamon over before covering with a bandage. However, as some people may be allergic to cinnamon and develop a rash after use, only small amounts should be used at any time to minimise any adverse reaction to the spice.

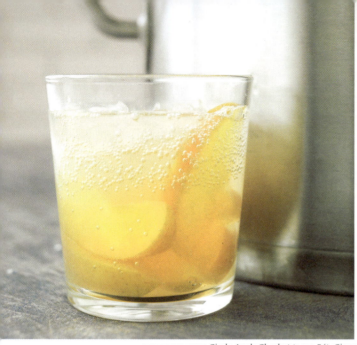
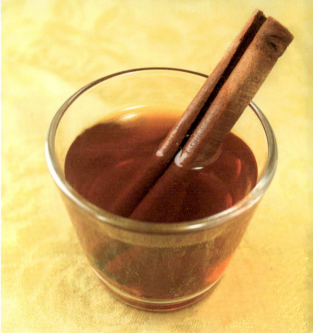

FROM LEFT TO RIGHT: Simla Apple Sharbat (page 54), Cinnamon Ginger Tea (page 54) OPPOSITE: Chettinad Masala Mutton (page 55)

Simla Apple Sharbat

Preparation time: 5 minutes
Cooking time: 2 minutes
Serves: 8

Ginger 5 thin slices

Cinnamon sticks 2, about 4-cm (2-in) long

Water 1 litre (32 fl oz / 4 cups)

Red apples 4, cored and sliced

Honey 60 ml (2 fl oz / ¼ cup), or to taste

Soda water 500 ml (16 fl oz /2 cups)

Ice cubes or crushed ice as required

Put all ingredients except soda water and ice into a pot and boil for 5 minutes.

Remove cinnamon sticks from pot and leave liquid to cool, then refrigerate until ready to serve.

Just before serving, add soda water and ice cubes or crushed ice to make a refreshing drink.

Cinnamon Ginger Tea

Cinnamon and ginger are highly complementary ingredients in this tea for the relief of morning sickness or nausea.

Water 1 litre (32 fl oz / 4 cups)

Ginger 3 peeled slices

Cinnamon sticks 2, about 4-cm (2-in) long

Tea leaves 1 Tbsp

Put water, ginger and cinnamon together in a pot and boil for 10 minutes.

Remove from heat and add tea leaves. Steep for 3 minutes. Strain and serve tea as it is, or with milk if desired.

Remedy for Phlegmy Cough

This remedy is good for removing phelgm if you have a phlegmy cough.

Ground cinnamon ½ tsp

Ground ginger ½ tsp

Ground cloves ¼ tsp

Honey 2 tsp

Boiling water 250 ml (8 fl oz / 1 cup)

Stir to mix all ingredients together and drink once a day until cough subsides.

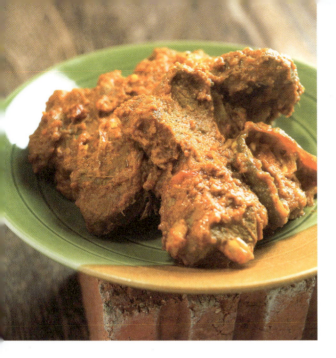

Chettinad Masala Mutton

Preparation time: 2 hours
Cooking time: 40 minutes
Serves: 8

Lean mutton cubes
  or mutton chops 1 kg (2 lb 3 oz)

Cooking oil 4 Tbsp

Cinnamon sticks 2, about 4-cm
  (2-in) long

Cardamoms 10

Cloves 8

Bay leaves 3

Star anise 1

Onions 3, large, peeled and chopped

Green chillies 3, slit lengthwise

Curry leaves 2 sprigs, stems discarded

Water 1.5 litres (48 fl oz / 6 cups)

Salt 1³/₄ tsp

Ground almond 5 Tbsp

Chopped coriander
  (cilantro) leaves 3 Tbsp

Marinade

Turmeric powder 1 tsp

Chilli powder 4 Tbsp

Coriander powder 3 Tbsp

Cinnamon powder 1 tsp

Natural yoghurt 200 ml
  (6²/₃ fl oz / ³/₄ cup)

Ginger paste 4 Tbsp

Garlic paste 5 Tbsp

Place mutton and marinade ingredients into a large bowl and combine well. Leave to marinate for 2 hours.

Heat oil in a pan and fry cinnamon, cardamoms, cloves, bay leaves and star anise until aromatic.

Add onions, green chillies and curry leaves and sauté until onions turn golden brown.

Add marinated mutton to pan and stir over very low heat until oil separates and mutton changes colour.

Add water and bring to the boil over medium heat for about 20 minutes.

Add salt, ground almond and coriander leaves and simmer until gravy thickens and mutton is tender. Serve with rice or bread.

clove

Common Cloves
Sanskrit Lavanga, Shriisanjnan
Tamil Graambu, Krambu, Karambu
Botanical Syzygium aromaticum

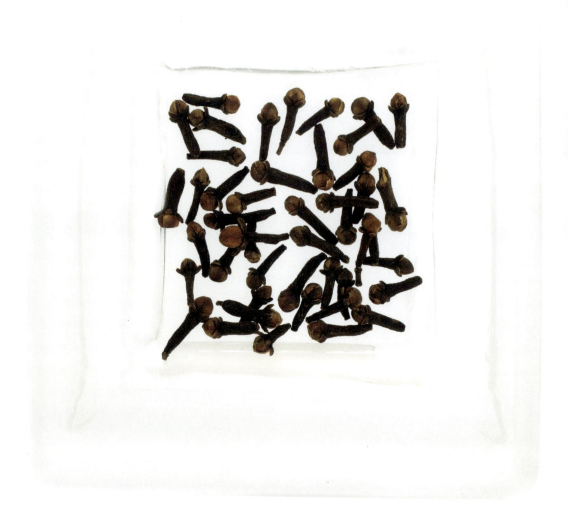

Clove trees grow all over India but are cultivated mainly in Kerala. The dried, rusty-brown flower buds which resemble small nails are known as cloves and are used extensively as spice while clove oil is extracted from the buds, leaves and stems of the tree. In India, both the clove oil and flower buds have been valued for their use in herbal remedies since ancient times.

Because of their warm, sweet and pungent flavour, cloves are used in an assortment of Indian recipes including meat dishes, *garam masala* and sweets. According to Indian herbal traditions, cloves act as an astringent, a stimulant, an appetite-enhancer, an anodyne and an aid to digestion. The spice is reputed to be effective in the treatment of respiratory and digestive conditions including asthma, coughs, tuberculosis, colic and nausea.

Clove essential oil contains mild anaesthetic and strong germicidal properties. It is an important ingredient in mouthwash and gargle for sore throats. It is also used to treat toothaches. Some dentists use clove oil as an oral anaesthetic as well as a disinfectant for root canals. Other uses of clove oil include external applications for poisonous bites, swellings and cuts.

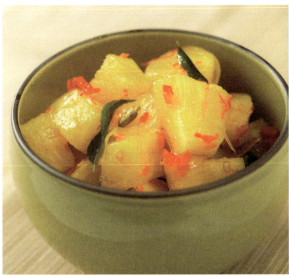 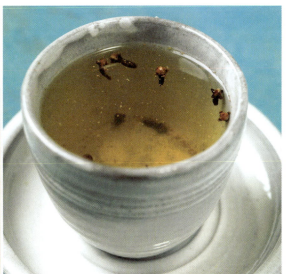

FROM LEFT TO RIGHT: *Pineapple Pachadi (page 57), Sleep Tea (page 58)*

Pineapple Pachadi

Preparation time: 10 minutes
Serves: 6
Cooking time: 5 minutes

Cooking oil 2 Tbsp

Cinnamon sticks 2, 3-cm (1¹/₂-in) long each

Cloves 7

Cardamoms 4

Red chillies 3, pounded

Onion 1, medium, peeled and sliced

Curry leaves 2 sprigs, stems discarded

Turmeric powder 1 tsp

Caster (superfine) sugar 60 g (2 oz)

Salt 1¹/₂ tsp

Ripe pineapple 1, large, peeled, cored and cut into small chunks

Heat oil and fry cinnamon, cloves and cardamoms until aromatic.

Add chillies, onion and curry leaves and sauté until aromatic.

Add remaining ingredients and stir-fry over high heat until pineapple is cooked but not right through. Remove and serve with rice and other dishes.

Sleep Tea

Cloves 1 tsp

Distilled water 250 m (8 fl oz /1 cup)

Honey 1 tsp

Boil cloves and water for about 4 minutes.

Strain liquid immediately. Add honey and stir until dissolved.

Drink about 1 hour before bedtime.

Clove Laddu

Preparation time: 15 minutes
Cooking time: 15 minutes
Serves: 6

Coarse semolina 400 g (14 oz)

Ghee (clarified butter) 4 Tbsp

Freshly grated coconut 300 g (10^1/$_2$ oz)

Cashew nuts 100 g (3^1/$_2$ oz), chopped

Raisins 100 g (3^1/$_2$ oz)

Cardamom powder 1 tsp

Clove powder ^{1}/$_2$ tsp

Icing sugar 300 g (10^1/$_2$ oz), sifted

Milk 60 ml (2 fl oz / ^{1}/$_4$ cup)

Place semolina and 2 Tbsp ghee into a non-stick pan and stir-fry over low heat until mixture turns light brown. Transfer to a mixing bowl.

In the same pan, add grated coconut and stir-fry over low heat until coconut turns light brown. Transfer to mixing bowl.

Heat remaining ghee in pan and fry cashew nuts until golden brown. Drain and transfer to mixing bowl.

In the same pan, fry raisins until they puff up. Drain and transfer to mixing bowl. Discard remaining ghee in pan.

Add cardamom and clove powders and icing sugar to mixture in mixing bowl. Sprinkle milk all over the mixture and combine well.

When mixture is slightly moist, take 1–2 Tbsp mixture in your hands, roll into a ball and place onto a large plate. Repeat until mixture is used up.

Set aside for 15 minutes until laddu balls become firm. Store in an airtight container. Serve as a snack.

Note: If too much milk is added to the mixture, the laddu balls will not become firm as the mixture is too wet. Therefore, sprinkle milk over the mixture as you combine the mixture to ensure that just enough milk is added to achieve a moist texture.

Soothing Bath

If you feel hot and slightly numb all over after having this bath, it means that the cloves have a sedative effect on you. However, staying in the bath for more than 30 minutes might induce up to 12 hours of slumber. If you do not wish for a long rest, then get out of the tub after not more than 30 minutes, dry off and crawl into bed.

Water 20 litres

Clove powder 2 Tbsp

Mix water and clove powder in a large pot and bring to the boil.

Pour into bath tub. Add cold water to adjust water to desired temperature.

Soak in tub and relax, and preferably drink one cup of sleep tea (see above recipe) to enhance the sedative effect of the cloves. If preferred, 3–4 drops of clove essential oil can be added to the bath water.

Note: Pregnant women should not use clove essential oil as the oil can stimulate the uterine muscles and trigger premature births.

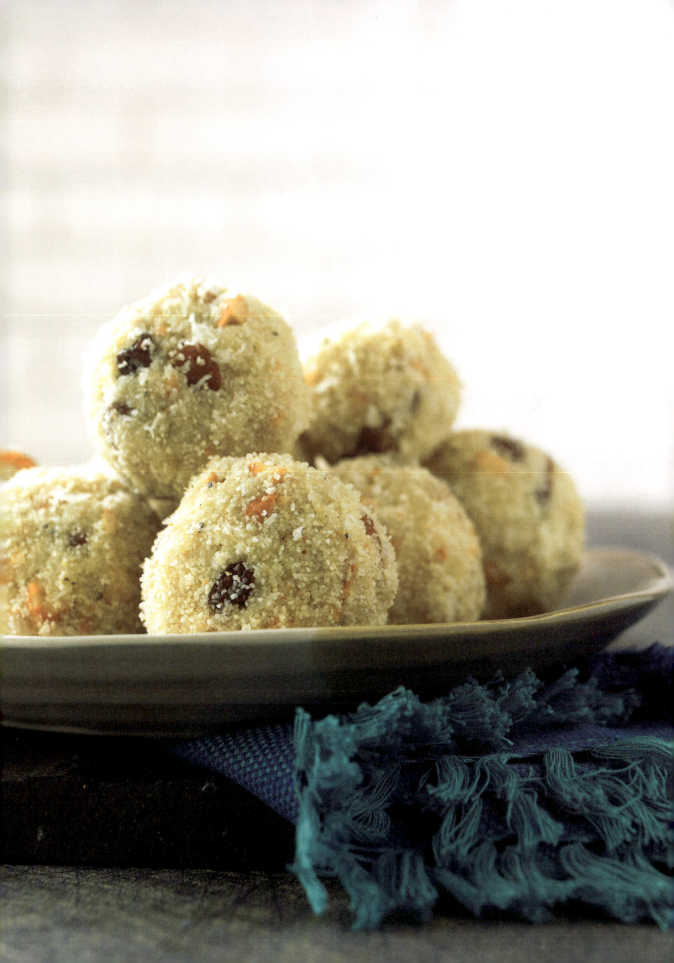

Coconut

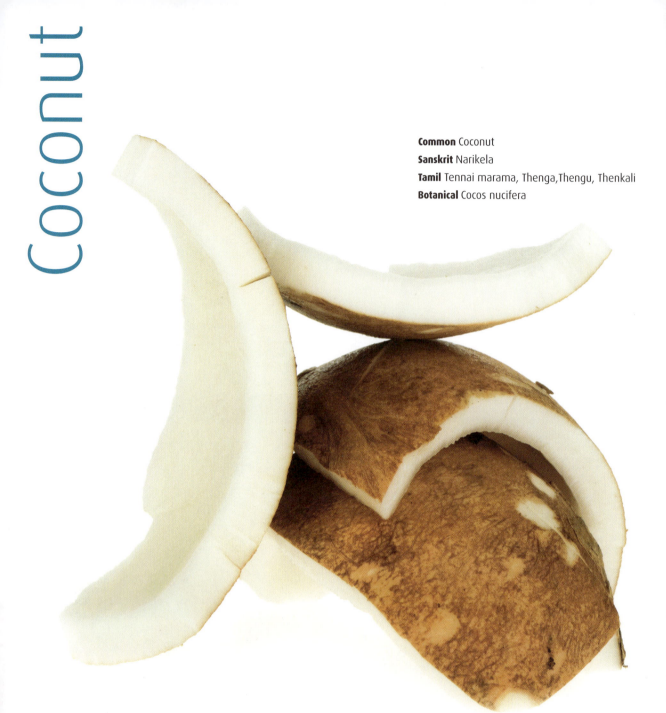

Common Coconut
Sanskrit Narikela
Tamil Tennai marama, Thenga, Thengu, Thenkali
Botanical Cocos nucifera

Cultivated in many tropical regions around the world, coconuts range from round to oblong in shape. The seeds which contain edible white flesh and a refreshing liquid are encased within thick, fibrous husks. In India, the coconut is regarded as a holy food. According to local legend, the fruit is a gift from the Hindu gods to human beings.

The usefulness of the coconut is apparent in the many forms in which the fruit is available, including fresh and dried coconut flesh, juice, cream, milk and oil. The juice and flesh of young, tender coconuts are often consumed right off the shells. Rich in B vitamins and minerals, the refreshing juice and tender sweet flesh are nutritious and alkaline in nature, thus aiding digestion. The juice of young to middle-aged coconuts is also regarded as an excellent remedy for flatulence, colitis, gastric ulcers, piles and urinary disorders. Avoid choosing mature coconuts with firm flesh and little juice for treatment as the firm flesh can lead to indigestion and instead cause hyperacidity.

In Indian cooking, freshly grated coconut flesh is often added to thicken the gravy of dishes, squeezed to extract coconut milk and used to prepare confectionery including coconut candies, cakes and breads. Grated or shredded coconut is also available in the dried form and serves as a substitute when freshly grated coconut is unavailable. However, use freshly grated coconut whenever possible as its flavour is infinitely superior to its dried counterpart.

Coconut oil is rich in lauric acid (the only other abundant source being human breast milk), which is considered responsible for the anti-viral, anti-microbial and anti-fungal properties present in the oil. Excellent for healing wounds and sunburn, coconut oil also moisturises the skin and hair; it is is widely employed in cosmetics and shampoos as well as natural beauty remedies including hair masks and moisturisers. As a cooking oil, the highly heat-resistant virgin coconut oil has been touted as one of the healthiest dietary oils on earth; its content of lauric acid help create a healthy digestive tract to facilitate better digestion and absorption of the nutrients in our food. Many recent medical studies have also indicated the efficacy of the oil in reducing the risk of cancer, diabetes and osteoporosis.

FROM LEFT TO RIGHT: *Surul Appam (page 62), Chocolate Coconut Candy (page 62)*

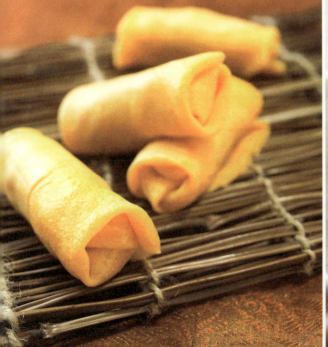
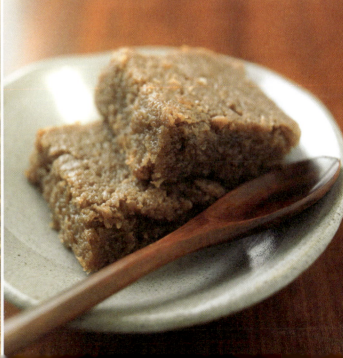

Surul Appam

Preparation time: 20 minutes
Cooking time: 20 minutes
Serves: 7

Filling

Grated coconut 200 g (7 oz)

**Grated palm sugar
(*gula melaka*)** 150 g (5^1/$_3$ oz)

Salt ^{1}/$_4$ tsp

Cardamom powder ^{1}/$_2$ tsp

Pancake Batter

Plain (all-purpose) flour
300 g (10^1/$_2$ oz), sifted

Salt 1 tsp

Eggs 2, medium, lightly beaten

Milk powder 2 Tbsp

Thin coconut milk 750 ml
(24 fl oz / 3 cups) (see page 50)

Egg-yellow food colouring ^{1}/$_2$ tsp

Cooking oil for brushing

Prepare filling. Put all ingredients into a frying pan and cook over low heat, stirring occasionally until filling is thoroughly combined and almost dry. Set aside.

Prepare pancakes. Put all ingredients for pancake batter except cooking oil into a mixing bowl. Mix well to remove any lumps in batter.

Heat a hot plate or non-stick pan and brush lightly with oil.

Pour in 1 ladleful (about 6 Tbsp) prepared batter and spread out thinly with the back of ladle. Cook until batter is firm on the underside, then turn over to cook the other side. Transfer cooked pancake to a plate and repeat until all batter is used up.

Place 1–2 Tbsp filling in the centre of each pancake, tuck in the sides and roll up into a tight roll. Repeat until all filling is used up. Serve at room temperature as a dessert or snack.

Chocolate Coconut Candy

Preparation time: 10 minutes
Cooking time: 20 minutes
Serves: 8

Freshly grated coconut 1 kg (2 lb 3 oz)

Caster (superfine) sugar 900 g
(1lb 15^1/$_2$ oz)

Condensed milk 2 cans

Butter 30 g (1 oz)

Salt ^{1}/$_4$ tsp

Cocoa powder 30 g (1 oz), dissolved
in 50 m (1^2/$_3$ fl oz/ ^{1}/$_4$ cup) water

Vanilla essence 2 tsp

Rice flour 30 g (1 oz)

Put all ingredients into a wok and cook over low heat, stirring constantly until mixture comes together into a thick, sticky mass and leaves sides of pan cleanly, or until a teaspoonful of mixture forms a soft ball when dropped into a glass of iced water.

Divide mixture between 2 greased 18 x 27-cm lamington trays.

Press mixture firmly into trays with the back of a metal spoon. Place a sheet of cling film (plastic wrap) on top of mixture and smoothen surface with the back of a metal spoon or roll over with a small rolling pin. Leave to set and cool.

When cool, cut into squares and serve as a sweet.

Herbal Coconut Hair Oil

Many women in Kerala have lustrous, long and thick hair. And one reason is that they massage their scalps with this oil daily.

Pure coconut oil 300 ml
(10 fl oz / 1^1/$_4$ cups), warmed

Hibiscus powder 2 Tbsp

Henna powder 1 Tbsp

Dried curry leaves 2 sprigs,
stems discarded

Place all ingredients into a sterilised glass bottle. Cover tightly and shake to mix well. Store for 3 months before using.

To use, rub 1–2 Tbsp oil into hair and scalp. Wrap head with a small bath towel for ^{1}/$_2$–1 hour.

Rinse off and shampoo hair as per normal.

Note: This oil keeps well for up to one year at room temperature.

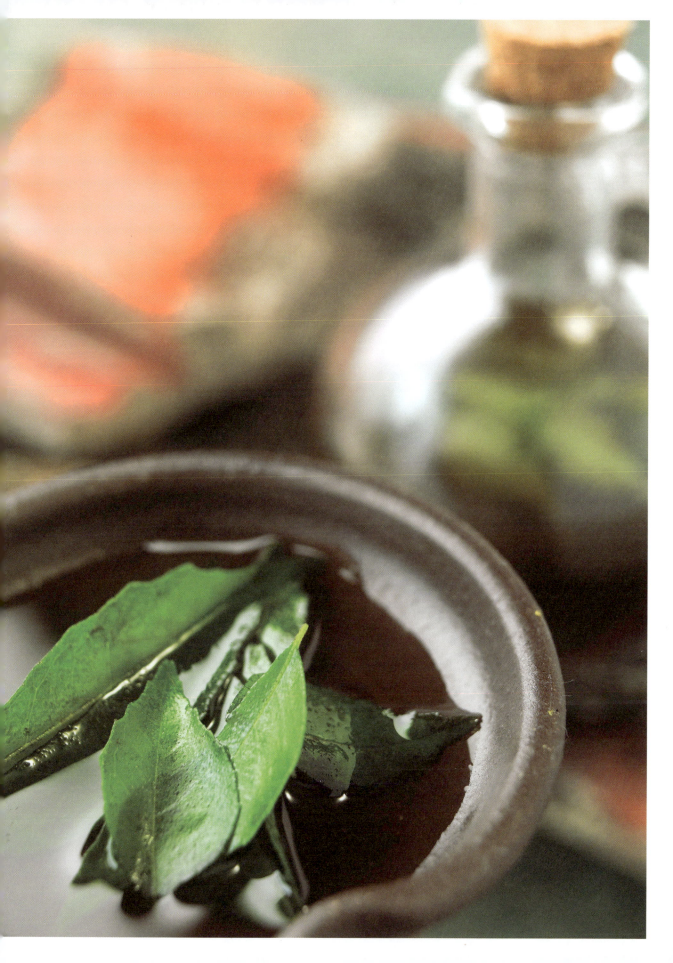

Cumin

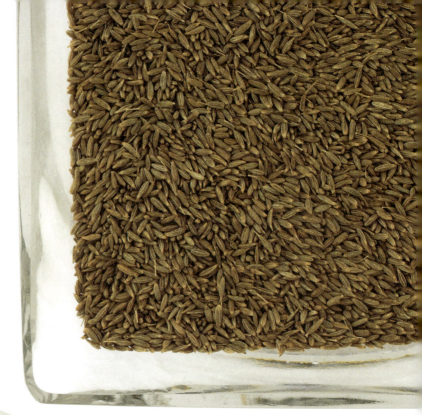

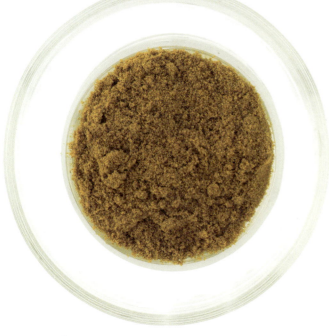

Common Cumin, Roman caraway
Sanskrit Jiraka, Ajaji, Jirana, Svetajiraka
Tamil Jirakam (Jeerakam), Cirakam
Botanical Cuminum Cyminum

Cumin seeds are oblong-shaped, longitudinally ridged, and yellowish-brown in colour. Although the small cumin seed looks rather unassuming, it more than compensates with an intense flavour which can be described as penetrating and peppery, with slight citrus overtones.

In India, cumin seeds are added to food preparations either as whole seeds or in powder form. Cumin is also a main ingredient in many Indian spice mixtures and curry powders. As with many other seed spices, cumin seeds should be lightly roasted to bring out the aroma before they are ground or used whole.

In traditional Indian healing, cumin seeds are boiled in water or used in conjunction with other herbs and ingredients such as rock salt or rock sugar to treat many common ailments. Adding a mixture of cumin seeds boiled with water to the bath helps cure skin rashes while eating cumin seeds with rock sugar aids in relieving piles. It is believed that cumin seeds are highly beneficial to the heart and digestive system. Cumin is also taken by Indian women who are breastfeeding to increase lactation. However, pregnant ladies should seek medical advice before using the spice as excess consumption may stimulate the uterine muscles and lead to spontaneous abortion.

With antibacterial properties, cumin seeds are natural breath fresheners and effective in healing mouth ulcers. Cumin is valuable in the treatment of insomnia; to induce sleep, mix one teaspoonful of roasted cumin powder with a mashed banana and consume this mixture before bedtime.

Cumin Tea

Cumin tea reduces body aches and acts as a natural sleep aid for those who have difficulty falling asleep. Since cumin tea has antiseptic properties, it is also effective for treating common cold and fever. To soothe a sore throat, add $1/2$ teaspoon ground ginger to the tea.

Cumin seeds 2 tsp, coarsely pounded

Water 350 ml (11 $^2/_3$ fl oz / 1 $^3/_8$ cups)

Put cumin seeds in a small heatproof bowl. Bring water to the boil and pour over cumin seeds. Steep for 5 minutes. Strain liquid and drink immediately.

Alternatively, boil cumin seeds and water together for a stronger-tasting tea, then strain and drink throughout the day.

Jeera Rice

Preparation time: 10 minutes
Cooking time: 15 minutes
Serves: 4

Ghee (clarified butter) 2 Tbsp

Cinnamon sticks 2, 3-cm (1 $^1/_2$-in) long each

Cloves 8

Cardamoms 8

Bay leaves 2

Black peppercorns $1/2$ tsp

Dried chillies 3, cut into 3-cm (1 $^1/_2$-in) pieces

Cumin seeds 2 tsp

Basmati rice 500 g (1lb 1 $^1/_2$ oz), washed and drained

Water 1 litre (32 fl oz / 4 cups)

Salt 1 $^1/_2$ tsp

Heat ghee and fry cinnamon sticks, cloves, cardamoms and bay leaves until very aromatic.

Add peppercorns, dried chillies and cumin seeds and fry until chillies turn a shade darker.

Add rice and stir-fry for a few seconds. Remove from heat and transfer to a rice cooker. Add water and salt, then stir to mix well. Switch on rice cooker.

When rice is cooked, serve with curry and vegetables.

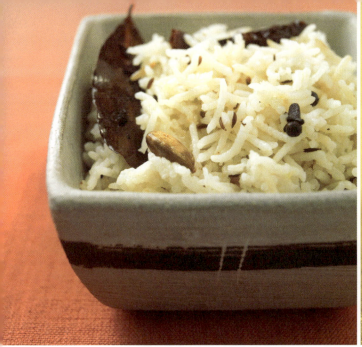
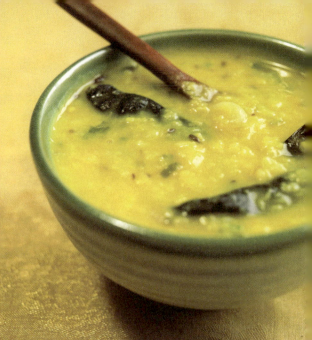

FROM LEFT TO RIGHT: Jeera Rice (page 65), Dhal Maharani (page 66) OPPOSITE: *Remedy for Swelling Gums (page 66)*

Dhal Maharani

Preparation time: 10 minutes
Cooking time: 15 minutes
Serves: 6

Skinned mung (green) beans (*moong* **dhal**) 250 g (9 oz), washed and drained

Ghee (clarified butter) 7 tsp

Turmeric powder 1 tsp

Green chillies 3, sliced

Garlic 4 cloves, peeled and minced

Water 750 ml (24 fl oz/ 3 cups)

Salt 1 1/2 tsp

Cumin powder 1 tsp

Cumin seeds 2 tsp

Dried chillies 2, cut into 3-cm (1 1/2-in) pieces

Onion 1, peeled and thinly sliced

Curry leaves 2 sprigs

Asafoetida powder 1/2 tsp

Chopped coriander (cilantro) leaves 2 Tbsp

Put mung beans, 1 tsp ghee, turmeric powder, chillies, garlic and water into a pan and boil until mung beans are cooked and mushy. Add salt and cumin powder and continue to boil.

Heat remaining ghee in a separate pan. Fry cumin seeds and dried chillies until aromatic and chillies turn brown.

Add onion, curry leaves and asafoetida powder. Sauté until onion turns golden brown. Transfer to mung bean mixture and stir to mix well.

Cook for another 2 minutes. Stir in chopped coriander leaves, remove from heat and serve hot with rice and other dishes.

Remedy for Swelling Gums

Cumin seeds 30 g (1 oz)

Rock salt 30 g (1 oz)

Dry-roast cumin seeds until aromatic. Cool before pounding together with rock salt.

To help reduce swelling of gums, place a little mixture (about 20 g / 2/3 oz) onto a finger and massage affected area in a light, circular motion.

Note: For convenience, grind more of the mixture and store in an airtight container for future use.

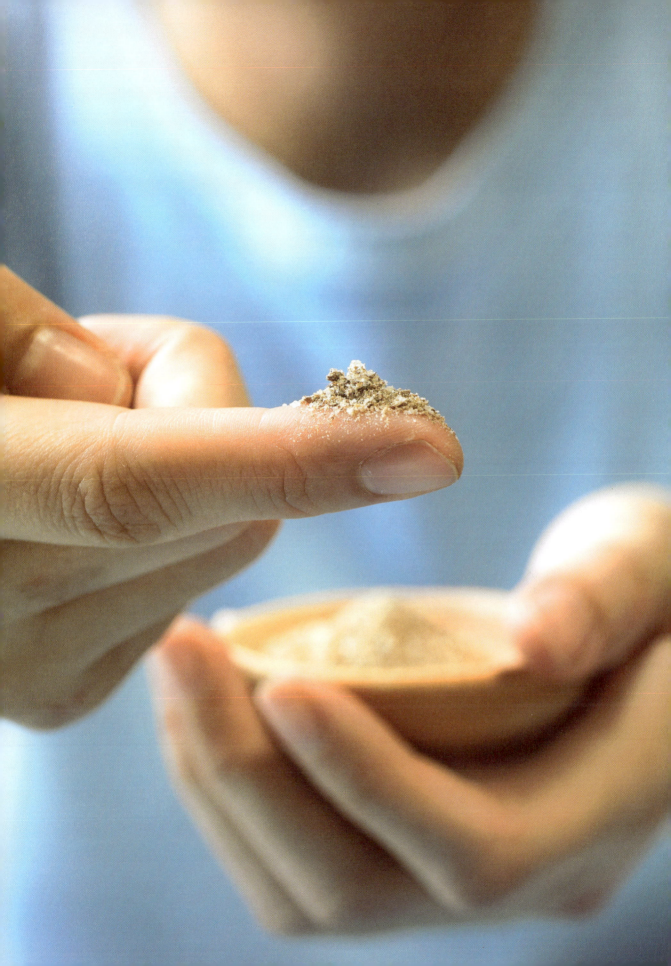

Curry Leaf

Common Curry leaves
Sanskrit Kaidarya, Saurabh nimb, Krishna nimba
Tamil Karuvapilai, Kariveppallai
Botanical Murraya koenigii

Used extensively in South India, curry leaves were introduced to countries such as Malaysia, Singapore and South Africa by South Indian immigrants. In Indian cooking, curry leaves are used to flavour a wide selection of fish and meat dishes as well as breads, and are an important ingredient in South Indian vegetarian cuisine. Curry-leaf chutney, a popular vegetarian dish in South India, is prepared by grinding curry leaves with coconut and spices. An excellent appetite-stimulant, the chutney is a good accompaniment to any meal.

A good source of calcium, phosphorus, iron and vitamin C, curry leaves are available either fresh or dried. Hanging from thin stems, the long, slender leaflets have a dark green-coloured surface with a paler shade of green on the underside. The leaves have a strong, warm and bitter-citrusy aroma when bruised or heated.

Curry leaves are used extensively in traditional Indian healing. The leaves and stems of the curry-leaf plant are believed to have tonic and carminative properties. Curry leaves are used to strengthen gastrointestinal functions; a drink of buttermilk mixed with a small amount of fresh curry-leaf juice acts as a mild laxative for curing constipation. Fresh curry-leaf juice mixed with lemon juice and sugar serves as another home remedy for treating indigestion. For the treatment of morning sickness, nausea and vomiting due to indigestion and an over intake of fats, a drink of curry-leaf juice mixed with lime juice is recommended.

The antiseptic properties of curry leaves make them useful for external treatments; poultices made with curry leaves can be applied on burns, bruises and skin rashes. Apart from being used in food and healing remedies, curry leaves are also used in many Indian beauty treatments. It is believed that the liberal consumption of curry leaves in one's diet will arrest the premature graying of hair. In many Indian villages, coconut oil boiled with curry leaves, is strained and massaged into the scalp to prevent excessive hair loss, promote hair growth and retain natural hair pigmentation. Some Indian ladies also concoct face masks using a mixture of curry leaves and turmeric powder to lighten dark spots on the face.

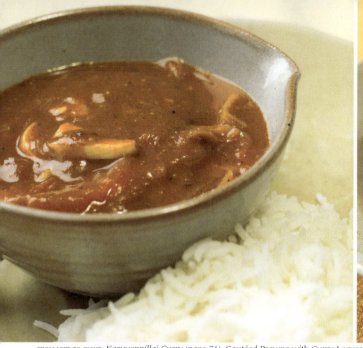
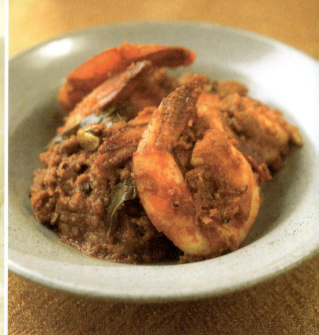

FROM LEFT TO RIGHT: Karuveppillai Curry (page 71), Sautéed Prawns with Curry Leaves (page 70) OPPOSITE: Remedy for Nausea and Vomiting (page 71)

Sautéed Prawns with Curry Leaves

Preparation time: 15 minutes
Cooking time: 15 minutes
Serves: 6

Cooking oil 2 Tbsp

Onion 1, peeled and sliced

Curry leaves 2 sprigs, stems discarded

Salt $1^1/_2$ tsp

Prawns (shrimps) 1 kg (2 lb 3 oz), medium, shelled and deveined

Spice Paste

Garlic 10 cloves, peeled

Ginger 2-cm (1-in) knob, peeled

Curry leaves 6 sprigs, stems discarded

Ripe tomatoes 2, medium, sliced

Shallots 100 g ($3^1/_2$ oz), peeled

Grated coconut 50 g ($1^2/_3$ oz)

Chilli powder 25 g (1 oz)

Coriander powder 1 tsp

Turmeric powder $^1/_2$ tsp

Cumin powder $^1/_2$ tsp

Garam masala 1 tsp

Water 400 ml ($13^1/_3$ fl oz / $1^5/_8$ cups)

Whole Spices

Cinnamon stick 1, 4-cm (2-in) long

Cardamoms 6

Cloves 4

Black mustard seeds $^1/_2$ tsp

Fennel seeds $^1/_2$ tsp

Black peppercorns 1 tsp

Blend (process) ingredients for spice paste until smooth. Set aside.

Heat oil and fry whole spices together until aromatic.

Add onion and curry leaves and sauté until onion turns golden brown.

Add spice paste and cook, stirring often until oil separates.

Add salt and prawns and stir-fry until prawns are cooked, and sauce has thickened. Remove and serve with rice or bread.

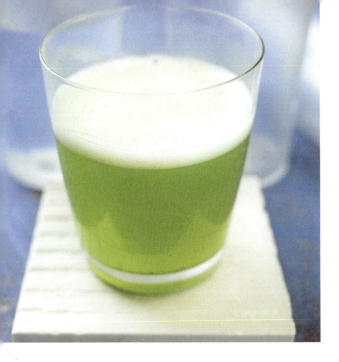

Remedy for Nausea and Vomiting

Curry leaves 30

Water 250 ml (8 fl oz / 1 cup)

Lemon juice 2 tsp

Honey 2 tsp

Blend (process) all ingredients together until smooth and drink to cure nausea.

Repeat this portion as required throughout the day.

Karuveppillai Curry

Preparation time: 15 minutes
Cooking time: 15 minutes
Serves: 5

Cooking oil 1 Tbsp

Dried chillies 15, cut into 2-cm (1-in) pieces

Split yellow lentils (*tur* dhal) 2 Tbsp

Black peppercorns 1$^1/_2$ Tbsp

White rice grains 1 Tbsp

Cumin seeds 1 Tbsp

Curry leaves 2 sprigs, stems discarded

Cooking oil 2 Tbsp

Black mustard seeds 1 tsp

Onion 1, medium, peeled and sliced

Garlic 6 cloves, peeled and sliced

Tomatoes 2, medium, diced

Tamarind pulp 120 g (4$^1/_2$ oz), mixed with 800 ml (26 fl oz / 3$^1/_4$ cups) water and strained

Salt 1$^1/_2$ tsp

Heat oil and fry chillies, lentils, peppercorns, rice, cumin seeds and curry leaves until aromatic and lentils turn golden brown. Remove from heat and leave aside to cool.

Using a coffee grinder, grind fried mixture into a powder. Set aside.

Heat oil and fry mustard seeds until they stop spluttering. Add onion and garlic and sauté until onion turns golden brown.

Add tomatoes and sauté until pulpy, then add tamarind juice, ground mixture and salt.

Boil for 10 minutes over low heat until gravy thickens and oil separates. Remove and serve hot with rice.

Date

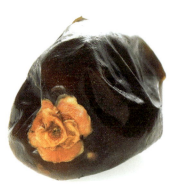 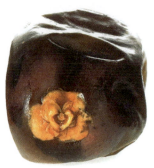 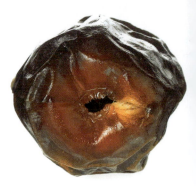

Common Date
Sanskrit Khajura
Tamil Karchuram, Perichchankay
Botanical Phoenix dactylifera

Dates are cultivated in countries such as Egypt, Saudi Arabia and India. The fruit of the date palm is oblong with an intensely sweet flesh. Ranging from yellow to reddish-brown in colour when fresh, it turns a dark brown colour when dried. Dates are widely used in Indian cooking, especially for making sweets, pickles and chutneys. A rich source of nutrients including vitamins A and B, protein, potassium and iron, dates are used in traditional Indian healing as a demulcent. Eating dates regularly helps establish friendly bacteria in the intestines for aiding digestion. They are effective as an expectorant to expel mucus in respiratory ailments as well as provide the roughage required to stimulate sluggish bowels for curing constipation. As a tonic food, dates are nourishing for the body and act as an excellent energy booster. To treat anaemia, take a blended drink of 300 ml (10 fl oz / 1¼ cups) milk with five dates every morning.

Date Halwa

Preparation time: 10 minutes
Cooking time: 15 minutes
Serves: 5

Pitted dates 400 g (14 oz)

Water 300 ml (10 fl oz / 1¼ cups)

Semolina 1 Tbsp

Grated jaggery 1 Tbsp

Ghee (clarified butter) 4 Tbsp

Roasted cashew nuts 100 g (3½ oz), chopped

Cardamom powder ½ tsp

Wash dates and soak in water for 1 hour. Blend (process) mixture to obtain a smooth paste.

Add mixture to a non-stick pan together with semolina, jaggery and ghee and cook, stirring constantly over low heat until mixture becomes a thick paste.

Add cashew nuts and cardamom powder and combine well.

Spoon halwa into a greased tray and spread mixture out evenly. Allow to cool before scooping serving portions onto small plates. Serve as a dessert.

Note: If a firmer texture is preferred, refrigerate halwa to set for a few hours then cut into desired shapes before serving.

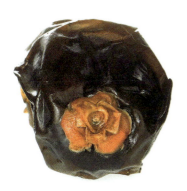
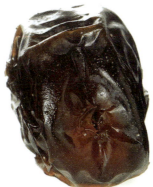
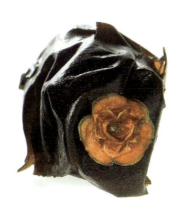

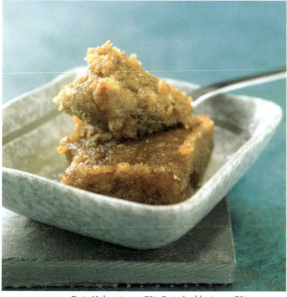
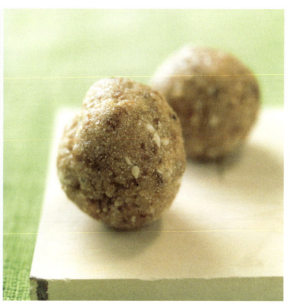

FROM LEFT TO RIGHT: Date Halwa (page 72), Date Laddu (page 73)

Date Laddu

Preparation time: 30 minutes
Cooking time: 10 minutes
Serves: 12

Pitted dates 200 g (7 oz), chopped to a paste-like consistency

Melted ghee (clarified butter) 1 Tbsp

Orange juice 100 ml (3$^1/_3$ fl oz / $^3/_8$ cup)

Caster (superfine) sugar 2 Tbsp

Fine semolina 80 g (3 oz)

White sesame seeds 150 g (5$^1/_3$ oz)

Cardamom powder $^1/_2$ tsp

Put dates, melted ghee, orange juice and sugar into a mixing bowl. Combine well to form a thick paste and set aside for 20 minutes.

Dry-roast fine semolina over low heat until aromatic and set aside. Dry-roast sesame seeds over low heat until aromatic, then grind into a coarse mixture.

Add semolina, ground sesame seeds and cardamom powder to paste and combine thoroughly. While mixture is still warm, use hands to shape into balls of about 2.5-cm (1-in) in diameter.

When cool, store laddu in an airtight container and refrigerate for at least 30 minutes to obtain a firmer texture before serving as a snack or dessert.

Note: It is important to shape laddu while the mixture is still warm, as the mixture will become too dry to shape into balls when cold.

Drumstick

Common Drumstick
Sanskrit Shigru, Shobhan jana
Tamil Murungai
Botanical Moringa oleifera

The Moringa tree is commonly known as the drumstick tree as it bears long pods of fruit which resemble drumsticks. Attached to thin stems, the leaves of the tree are small and oval, while its small, waxy and creamy white flowers bloom in clusters. Many parts of the tree are edible, including the leaves, flowers, bark and even roots.

Long regarded as a miracle tree by the Indians, scientific research has revealed drumstick leaves to be of exceptional nutritional value, containing very high levels of protein, potassium and calcium as well as vitamins A and C. While the leaves can be eaten raw, steamed, pickled, stir-fried or cooked in curries and soups, the tender green fruit pods are usually sliced and added to savoury and meat dishes.

In traditional medicine, the gum of the tree is used for external applications such as in the treatment of rheumatism and venomous bites as it has antiseptic properties, while oil pressed from the seeds is used to treat gout and rheumatism. The leaves and bark are often made into poultices for treating external wounds, skin problems and glandular swelling. Drumstick leaves are also believed to cleanse the blood, dispel phlegm and aid digestion when consumed. A common folk remedy for treating stomach ulcers involves taking ground drumstick leaves with yoghurt.

High-Calcium Tonic Drink

Children who drink this milk daily will have strong bones. This is also a good tonic for breast-feeding mothers as it increases lactation.

Drumstick leaves 50 g (2 oz)

Fresh cow's milk 300 ml
(10 fl oz / 1¹/₄ cups)

Boil drumstick leaves and milk together over low heat for 5 minutes.

Cool thoroughly, then strain and drink.

FROM LEFT TO RIGHT: High-Calcium Tonic Drink (page 75), Drumstick Leaf Bhajis (page 76)

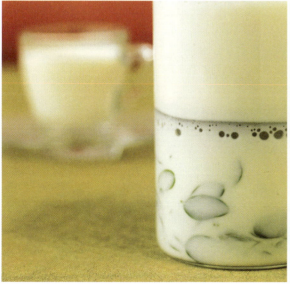
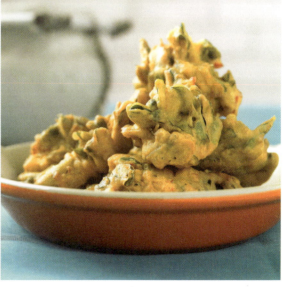

Drumstick Sothi

Preparation time: 15 minutes
Cooking time: 15 minutes
Serves: 6

Cooking oil 1¹/₂ Tbsp

Black mustard seeds 1 tsp

Fenugreek seeds ¹/₂ tsp

Cinnamon stick 1, 3-cm (1¹/₂-in) long

Onion 1, medium, peeled and sliced

Red chillies 2, slit lengthwise

Curry leaves 2 sprigs, stems discarded

Thin coconut milk 1.25 litres
(40 fl oz /5 cups) (see page 50)

Turmeric powder 1 tsp

Cumin powder 1 tsp

Salt 1¹/₂ tsp

Drumstick pods 6, cut into 4-cm
(2-in) pieces

Ripe tomatoes 2, sliced

Thick coconut milk 250 ml
(1 cup / 8 fl oz) (see page 50)

Lime juice 1¹/₂ Tbsp

Heat oil and fry mustard and fenugreek seeds and cinnamon stick until mustard seeds stop spluttering.

Add onion, red chillies and curry leaves and stir-fry until aromatic.

Add thin coconut milk, turmeric and cumin powders, salt, drumstick pieces and tomatoes.

Bring to the boil and cook for 10 minutes or until drumstick pods are tender.

Stir in thick coconut milk and bring to the boil for 1 minute. Remove from heat.

Stir in lime juice just before serving. Serve with rice and other dishes.

Drumstick Leaf Bhajis

Preparation time: 20 minutes
Cooking time: 15 minutes
Serves: 7

Garlic 3 cloves, peeled and
finely minced

Onions 2, medium, peeled and
finely chopped

Red chilli 1, finely chopped

Drumstick leaves 150 g (5 oz)

Cooking oil for deep-frying

Batter

Chickpea flour (besan) 250 g (9 oz)

Rice flour 4 Tbsp

Baking powder ¹/₂ tsp

Meat curry powder 2 tsp

Turmeric powder 1 tsp

Salt 1¹/₄ tsp

Ajwain seeds ¹/₂ tsp

Cumin seeds 1 tsp

Asafoetida powder ¹/₂ tsp

Water 300 ml (10 fl oz / 1¹/₄ cups)

Put all ingredients for batter into a mixing bowl and combine well.

Add all remaining ingredients except cooking oil and combine into a thick mixture. Set aside for 15 minutes.

Deep-fry tablespoonfuls of mixture in hot oil until golden brown, then drain on absorbent paper towels and serve hot as a snack.

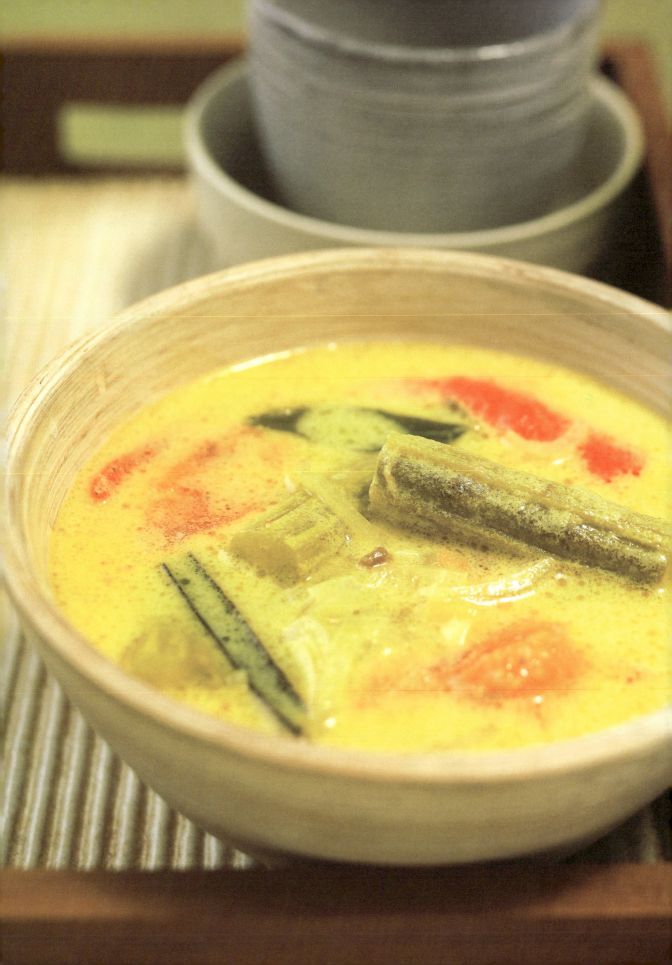

Fennel

Common Fennel
Sanskrit Shatapuspha, Madhurika
Tamil Perun siragum, Shombu, Sohikire
Botanical Foeniculum vulgare

Fennel has been known to traditional healers since time immemorial. It was believed to be the cure-all for people to stay young, strong and healthy.

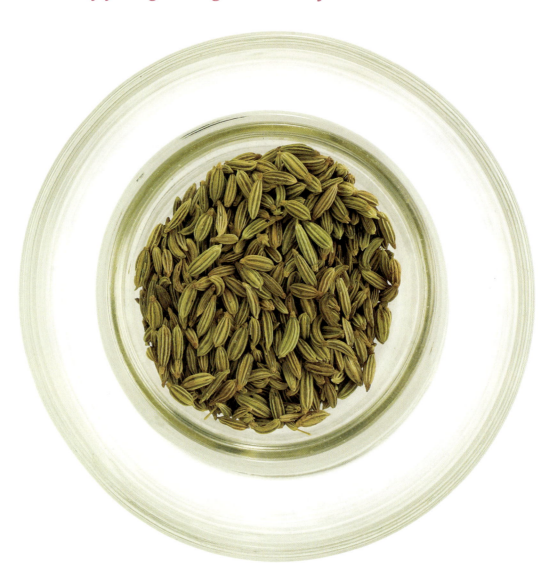

A long, thin seed that ranges from brown to light green in colour, the fennel seed has a warm and sweet aroma with a flavour similar to anise. It is an extremely versatile spice that is used to flavour a wide variety of foods including seafood and meat dishes, breads and desserts. Ground fennel also features as a key component in many Indian curry powder mixes. Fennel seeds are commonly used in India to add the sweetish and aromatic flavour of the spice to the making of medicines, liquors and perfumes.

In Indian natural healing traditions, fennel is known as a carminative and is especially effective in the treatment of gastrointestinal ailments. Fennel seeds are commonly offered for chewing at the end of a heavy Indian meal as a digestive and a natural mouth freshener. A gargle made by boiling fennel seeds in water helps to soothe sore throats as the spice contains antibacterial properties. Other applications of fennel include its use as an antidote for insect bites and food poisoning and as an appetite depressant to control weight gain.

Fennel oil, with its mildly anaesthetic properties, alleviates pain when rubbed on rheumatic joints. Fennel is also used as an ingredient in eye wash to relieve minor eye irritations.

Fennel Chai

Preparation time: 5 minutes
Cooking time: 5 minutes
Serves: 5

Fennel seeds 1 Tbsp
Cardamoms 5
Ginger 3 peeled slices
Water 1.5 litres (48 fl oz / 6 cups)
Tea leaves 2 Tbsp
Milk and sugar to taste

Using mortar and pestle, pound fennel seeds coarsely.

Put pounded fennel seeds, cardamoms, ginger, water and tea leaves into a pot and boil for 5 minutes.

To serve, strain tea and add milk and sugar to taste.

Facial Cleanser

Crushed fennel seeds 1¹/₂ Tbsp
Boiling water 250 ml (8 fl oz / 1 cup)
Honey 1 tsp
Yoghurt 1 Tbsp, whisked

Steep fennel seeds in boiling water. Set aside to cool.

When cool, add remaining ingredients and mix well.

Dip a piece of cotton wool into mixture and gently wipe all over face and neck. Repeat with fresh pieces of cotton wool.

Rinse face with cool water and pat dry with a clean towel.

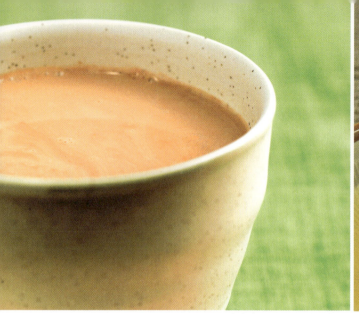
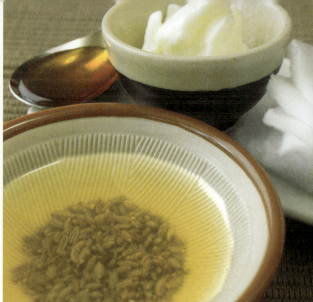

FROM LEFT TO RIGHT: Fennel Chai (page 79), Facial Cleanser (page 79), OPPOSITE: Fennel Brittle (page 80)

Fennel Brittle

Preparation time: 5 minutes
Cooking time: 10 minutes
Serves: 6

Fennel seeds 50 g (2 oz)

Caster (superfine) sugar 100 g
(3$^1/_2$ oz)

Water 2 Tbsp

Line a greased baking tray with non-stick baking paper. Set aside.

Dry-roast fennel seeds over low heat, stirring occasionally until lightly browned and aromatic.

Put sugar and water into a pan and cook over medium heat until sugar has dissolved. Continue to cook, stirring occasionally until sugar mixture has caramelised and turned golden-brown.

Remove from heat and quickly stir in fennel seeds. Immediately pour onto prepared baking tray and spread out with the back of a spoon before syrup hardens.

When brittle has cooled thoroughly and hardened, break into pieces and serve as a snack.

Fennel Flu Tea

This tea remedy is great for bringing relief for coughs and colds. For colicky babies, try soothing them by adding not more than 1-2 teaspoons of this infusion to the feed bottle.

Fennel seeds 1 tsp, coarsely pounded

Boiling water 250 ml (8 fl oz / 1 cup)

Honey to taste (optional)

Place fennels seeds in a cup. Pour boiling water over and leave to steep for 5 minutes.

Strain and stir in honey to taste, if desired, before drinking.

Fennel is widely regarded as a spice popular among women in India. Many Indian women take fennel to increase lactation when breastfeeding. Fennel is also useful for regulating the menstrual cycle and providing relief for menopausal symptoms. Fennel tea is a remedy commonly prescribed for the relief of menstrual cramps. If breastfeeding, soak a small, clean cotton towel in a warm fennel infusion and apply as a compress on sore nipples for up to three times a day. For minor skin infections, compresses can be applied for up to three times a day until the infections clear up. Drinking fennel tea infusion is also beneficial for adults suffering from excessive flatulence.

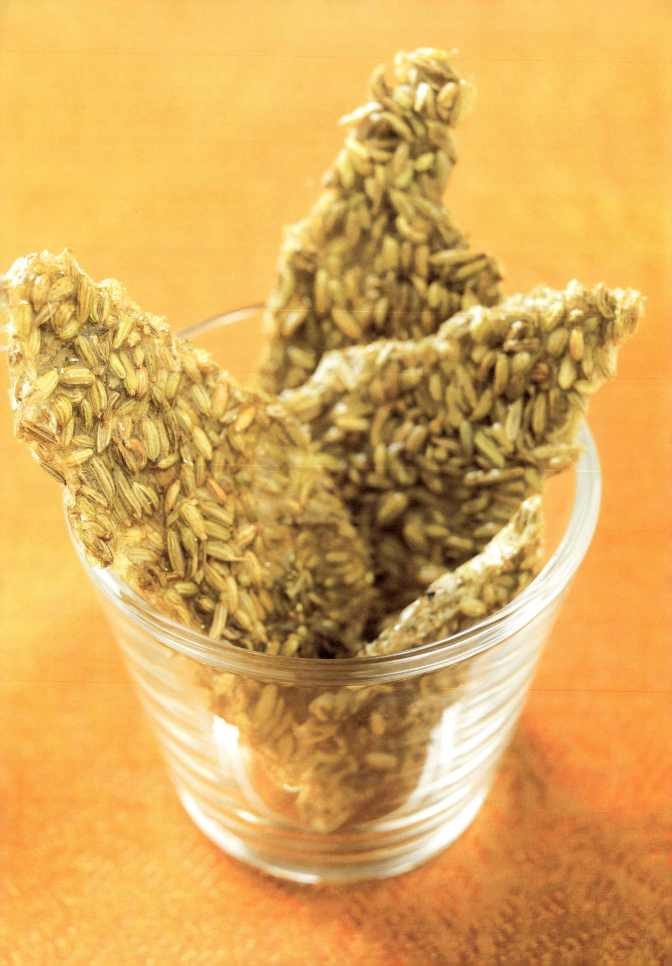

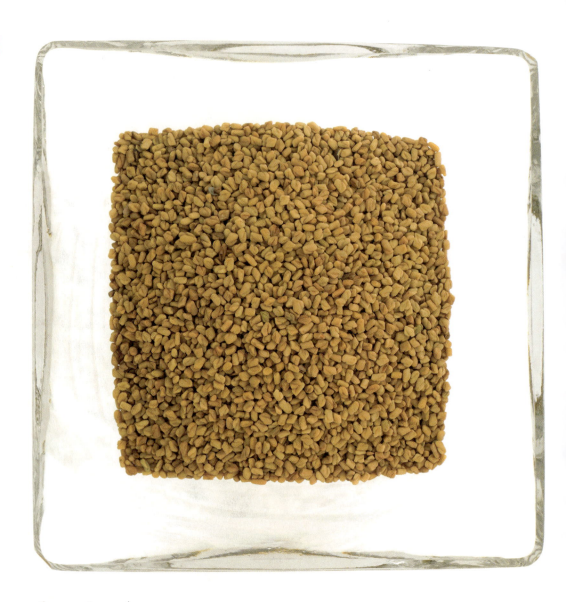

Common Fenugreek
Sanskrit Methika, Medhika, Chandrika
Tamil Meti, Vendayam, Vetani
Botanical Trigonella foenum-graecum

Fenugreek seeds are small, yellowish-brown in colour, furrowy and almost oblong in shape. Available whole or ground into a powder, dry-roast the seeds lightly before use, if you are using them whole, to release the strong, aromatic and bittersweet flavour of the spice.

In Indian cuisine, fenugreek is used in chutneys and pickles to add a tangy flavour. Ground roasted fenugreek seeds are used as a coffee substitute and in South India, fenugreek is an essential spice in cooking fish curry. Often ground and mixed with other spices, fenugreek is a common component of various curry powder mixes. Fenugreek leaves are also a delicacy in India and feature prominently in North Indian cuisine; dried fenugreek leaves are used for flavouring vegetables including potatoes, cabbages and turnips while fresh fenugreek leaves are added to cooked dishes including lentil stews and fritters, or consumed raw in salads.

For medicinal healing, fenugreek seeds are used as a carminative, for soothing the stomach and gastrointestinal tract while aiding digestion and dispelling wind at the same time. It is believed that fenugreek has aphrodisiac properties; it also serves as an anodyne, providing relief for menstrual cramps. Other treatments in which fenugreek is used include home remedies for reducing blood pressure and treating anaemia. In India, the use of fenugreek is traditionally encouraged among breastfeeding mothers to increase lactation. Fenugreek is also widely used in home remedies for the treatment of respiratory ailments because it helps to relieve congestion by removing excessive mucus and phelgm from the lungs, reduce inflammation and fight infection of the lungs.

The seeds are also used in many home beauty treatments. Fenugreek prevents the premature greying of hair and is used in hair masks. Soothing for skin eruptions, fenugreek is an excellent ingredient for making poultices to treat acne. It is effective in maintaining a smooth and silky skin and is an ingredient in natural facial masks.

Fenugreek Hair Mask

Try out this great recipe for glossy and silky hair.

Fenugreek seeds 2 Tbsp, soaked in water for 30 minutes and drained

Dried fenugreek leaves 2 Tbsp

Milk or coconut milk 200 ml (6²/₃ fl oz / ³/₄ cup) (see page 50)

Blend (process) all ingredients until smooth.

Apply paste onto pre-washed scalp and hair and leave on for 20 minutes.

Rinse off and shampoo as usual.

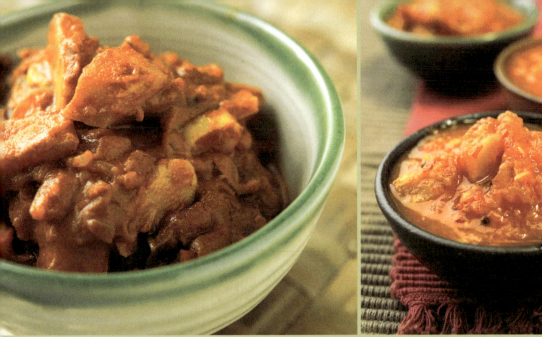

FROM LEFT TO RIGHT: Plantain Curry (page 84), Tomato Pickle (page 84) OPPOSITE: Fenugreek Beauty Mask (page 85)

Plantain Curry

Preparation time: 15 minutes
Cooking time: 15 minutes
Serves: 6

Cooking oil 2 Tbsp

Fennel seeds 1 tsp

Fenugreek seeds 2 tsp

Onion 1, large, peeled and thinly sliced

Garlic 5 cloves, peeled and sliced

Curry leaves 2 sprigs, stems discarded

Tomatoes 2, large, finely chopped

Tamarind pulp 150 g (5 $\frac{1}{3}$ oz), mixed with 1.5 litres (48 fl oz/ 6 cups) and strained

Salt $1\frac{1}{4}$ tsp

Plantains 4, large, peeled and cut into 1-cm ($\frac{1}{2}$-in) pieces

Dry Spices

Chilli powder $1\frac{1}{2}$ Tbsp

Coriander powder 4 Tbsp

Cumin powder 1 tsp

Turmeric powder 1 tsp

Heat oil and fry fennel and fenugreek seeds until aromatic.

Add onion, garlic and curry leaves and sauté until onions turn golden brown.

Add tomatoes and sauté until pulpy.

Add dry spices and tamarind juice and bring to the boil for 10 minutes.

Stir in salt and plantains. Boil until plantains are cooked through. Remove and serve hot with rice.

Gargle for Sore Throat

A gargle made from fenugreek seeds is effective for treating the occasional sore throat.

Fenugreek seeds 3 Tbsp

Mint leaves a handful

Water 1 litre (32 fl oz / 4 cups)

Boil fenugreek seeds and mint leaves in water for 15 minutes.

Strain liquid and cool.

Gargle with solution regularly until soreness of throat subsides.

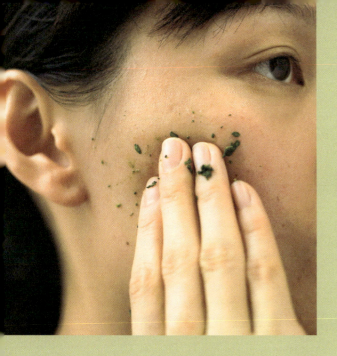

Fenugreek Beauty Mask

For younger-looking skin and clear complexion, try this formula.

Fenugreek seeds 2 Tbsp, soaked in
   water for 30 minutes and drained

Dried fenugreek leaves 2 Tbsp

Milk or coconut milk 200 ml
   (6 2/3 fl oz / 3/4 cup)

Chickpea flour (besan) 1 Tbsp

Blend (process) all ingredients together, except chickpea flour until smooth.

Add chickpea flour and stir until paste is lump-free.

Apply a thin layer onto clean and dry face and neck.

Leave on mask for 15 minutes or until dry. Rinse off with lukewarm water and pat dry with a clean towel.

Tomato Pickle

Preparation time: 10 minutes
Cooking time: 35 minutes
Makes: 6 x 250 ml jars

Gingelly oil 300 ml (10 fl oz / 1 1/4 cups)

Fenugreek seeds 1 Tbsp

Black mustard seeds 2 tsp

Turmeric powder 1 Tbsp

Slightly unripe tomatoes 1 1/2 kg
   (3 lb 4 1/2 oz), cubed

Salt 1 Tbsp

Sugar 1 Tbsp

Spice Blend

Dried chillies 25 g (1 oz), soaked for
   20 minutes and cut into pieces

Ginger 220 g (8 oz), peeled and sliced

Garlic 200 g (8 oz), peeled and left whole

Black mustard seeds 2 tsp

Rice vinegar 400 ml
   (13 1/3 fl oz / 1 5/8 cups)

Prepare spice blend. Blend (process) all ingredients together to obtain a coarse mixture. Set aside.

Heat oil in a deep pan, then add fenugreek and mustard seeds and fry until mustard seeds stop spluttering. Add remaining ingredients and spice blend.

Cook, stirring occasionally until pickle thickens. Remove from heat and set aside to cool thoroughly.

Store in sterilised glass jars and and set aside for 2 days before serving with rice and other dishes. If refrigerated, pickle can be kept for up to a year.

Galangal

Common Galangal, Greater galangal
Sanskrit Kulanja, Kulinjan
Tamil Arattai, Perattai
Botanical Alpinia galanga

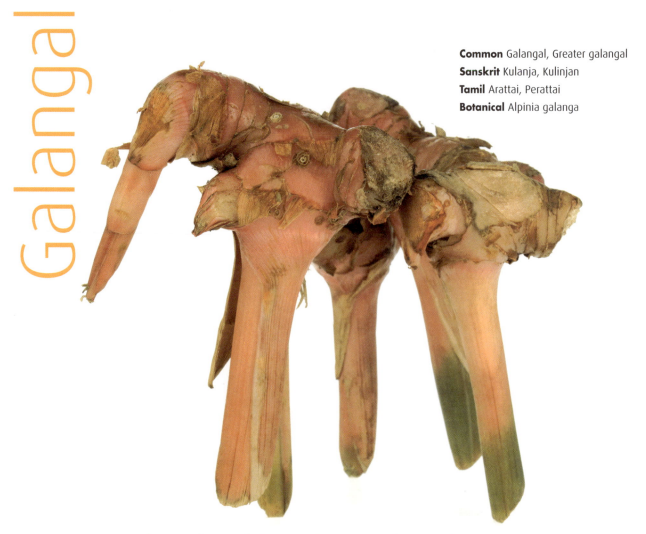

The galangal is a rhizome from the ginger family. It has an aromatic and mildly spicy flavour. Unlike ginger, galangal is tough and difficult to break, therefore use a strong, sharp knife when cutting the stem.

While fresh galangal has a distinctive flowery fragrance, dried galangal has a more spicy and sweetish-aromatic flavour that is similar to cinnamon. Both the fresh and dried galangal are used in a wide variety of Indian dishes. The fresh stem lends a wonderful aroma to dishes such as curries and chutneys and, like ginger, galangal goes well with garlic.

In traditional Indian healing practices, galangal is used for the treatment of nausea, stomach problems and catarrh. It is especially effective in curing flatulence and is also a natural remedy for seasickness. Its anti-inflammatory quality also lends well to its use in remedies for rheumatism. As a nervine tonic, galangal helps to stimulate the nervous system while its antibacterial property makes it useful in the treatment of persistent fevers.

Galangal Scrub

A facial or body scrub for smooth, glowing skin. Simply double or triple the quantity of ingredients for a full facial and body scrub.

Galangal 2-cm (1-in) knob, peeled and diced

Grated coconut 2 Tbsp

Chopped jaggery 2 tsp

Using mortar and pestle, pound all ingredients together to obtain a coarse mixture.

Rub all over face and body with gentle, circular motion.

Rinse off and shower as usual.

Galangal Milk Tea

This tea is effective in the treatment of nausea, diarrhoea and indigestion and can be drunk throughout the day.

Galangal 3 thin, peeled slices

Cardamoms 2

Black peppercorns 2

Water 400 ml (13$^1/_3$ fl oz (1$^5/_8$ cups)

Condensed milk 3 Tbsp

Using mortar and pestle, pound galangal, cardamoms and peppercorns coarsely.

Put pounded mixture and water into a pot and boil for 3 minutes.

Strain and stir in condensed milk just before serving.

Galangal Tea for Stomach-aches

Galangal 3-cm (1$^1/_2$-in) knob, peeled and thinly sliced

Water 500 ml (16 fl oz / 2 cups)

Boil all ingredients together for 5 minutes.

Strain tea and drink twice a day, about 1 cup (250 ml / 8 fl oz) each time.

FROM LEFT TO RIGHT: Galangal Milk Tea (page 87), Galangal Scrub (page 87)

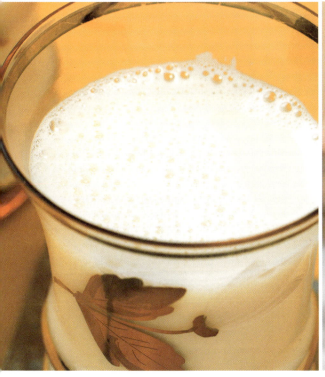
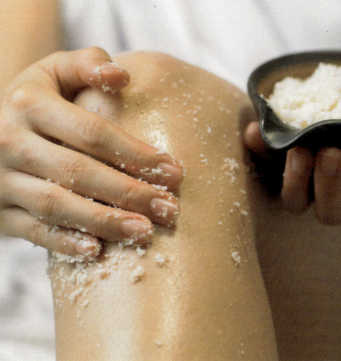

Garlic

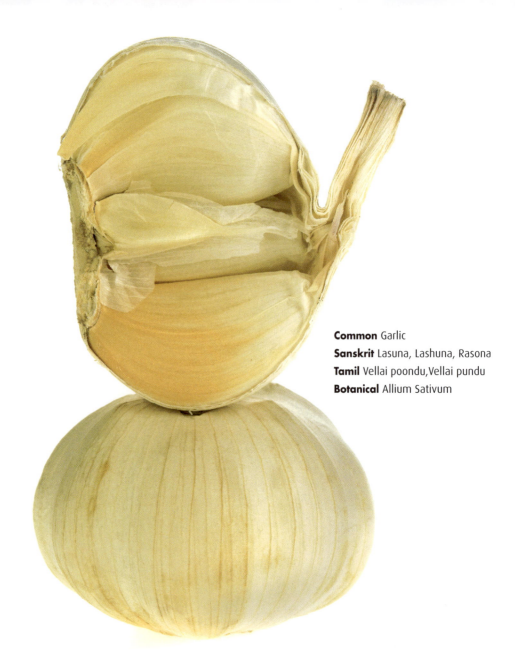

Common Garlic
Sanskrit Lasuna, Lashuna, Rasona
Tamil Vellai poondu, Vellai pundu
Botanical Allium Sativum

Garlic is well-known for its pungent odour and taste. It is completely safe for home use and is a powerful, natural treatment for many health problems. Garlic can be eaten raw or used in cooking. In fact, it is such a strong-tasting herb that some people simply rub the pot or utensil with a peeled clove of garlic to impart a more subdued flavour to the food.

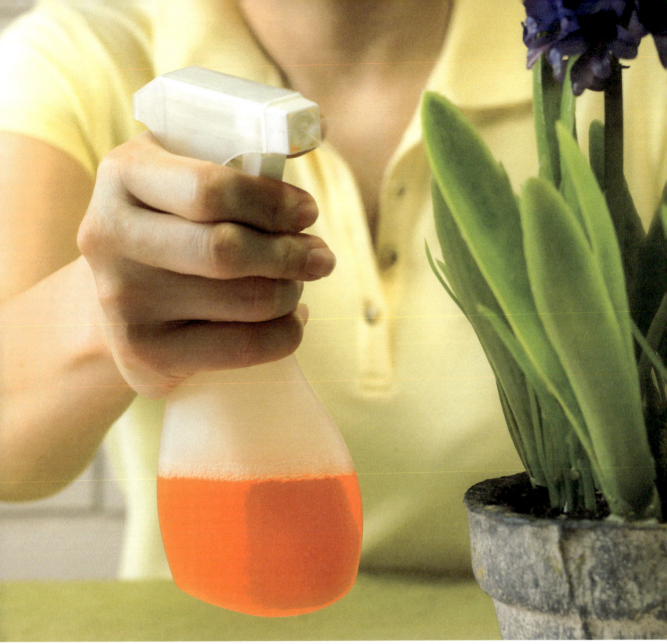

Natural Pest Repellent (page 91)

Garlic is believed to have carminative, antibacterial and antiviral properties. It is used to aid digestion, remove flatulence, purify the blood and kill worms in the stomach. For internal problems, eating garlic raw probably increases the efficacy of the treatment. For respiratory ailments including coughs, colds and sore throats, a common natural remedy involves steeping several cloves of garlic in half a cup of water overnight and drinking it in the morning. As garlic is an antiseptic, garlic oil is applied externally on festering wounds and sores to help speed up the healing process. In India, garlic is also used in folk remedies to treat insect stings and snake bites. As some studies have shown, the herb may help lower blood cholesterol levels by inhibiting the clogging of blood vessels which also help reduce blood pressure.

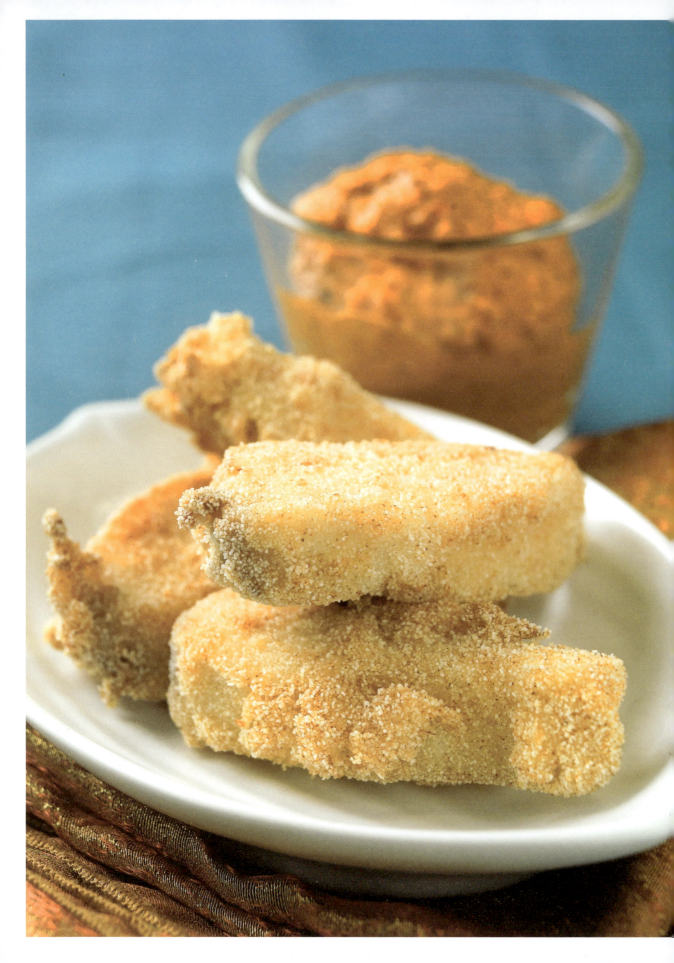

Natural Pest Repellent

Garlic 3 cloves, peeled
Chilli powder 1 Tbsp
Water 2 litres (64 fl oz / 8 cups)
Liquid soap 2 Tbsp

Using mortar and pestle, pound garlic coarsely.

Place garlic, chilli powder, water and liquid soap into a jug and stir to mix well.

Strain liquid and transfer to a spray bottle.

Spray at areas infested with ants, or plants attacked by aphids or ants. Prepare and use on the same day, discarding any leftover liquid.

Flu Remedy

This infusion of garlic cloves with antibacterial properties is effective in warding off coughs and colds.

Boiling water 500 ml (16 fl oz / 2 cups)
Garlic cloves 100 g (3¹/₂ oz), peeled and left whole
Fennel seeds ¹/₂ tsp
Honey to taste

Pour boiling water over garlic cloves and fennel seeds.

Set aside for 12 hours.

Strain liquid and stir in honey to taste. Drink twice daily, 250 ml (8 fl oz / 1 cup) each time.

Note: The garlic cloves can be reserved for cooking.

Garlic Fish Fingers

Preparation time: 20 minutes
Cooking time: 15 minutes
Serves: 4

Fish fillet 500 g (1 lb 1¹/₂ oz), cut into fingers
Ginger paste 1 Tbsp
Garlic paste 3 Tbsp
Salt 1 tsp
Lime juice 1 Tbsp
Semolina 100 g (3¹/₂ oz)
Chilli powder 2 tsp
Curry powder 1 tsp
Cooking oil for deep-frying

Marinate fish fingers with ginger and garlic paste, salt and lime juice in a large bowl. Set aside for 15 minutes.

In a separate bowl, mix semolina, chilli and curry powders together.

Coat marinated fish fingers in semolina mixture. Shake off any excess mixture and deep-fry fish fingers in hot oil until golden brown.

Drain on absorbent paper towels and serve hot with garlic chutney (see recipe below) as a snack.

Garlic Chutney

Preparation time: 10 minutes
Cooking time: 10 minutes
Serves: 6

Cooking oil 2 tsp
Garlic 5 cloves, peeled and sliced
Dried chillies 10, cut into 2-cm (1-in) pieces
Grated coconut 150 g (5¹/₃ oz),
Tamarind pulp 40 g (1¹/₂ oz), mixed with 200 ml (6²/₃ fl oz/ ³/₄ cup) water and strained
Salt 1 tsp

Heat oil and sauté garlic until lightly browned. Remove and set aside.

In same oil, sauté dried chillies and coconut until coconut turns a shade darker.

Blend (process) coconut mixture, garlic, tamarind juice and salt together until smooth.

Serve as a dip for fish fingers or other deep-fried foods.

Ghee

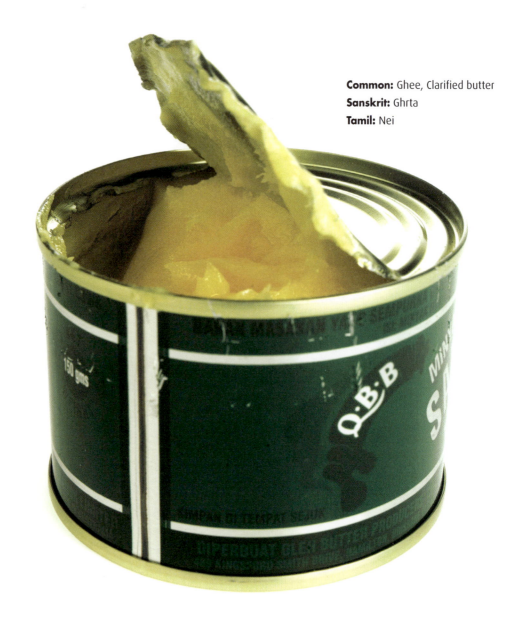

Common: Ghee, Clarified butter
Sanskrit: Ghrta
Tamil: Nei

Ghee is clarified butter that is lactose-free and does not contain any milk solids. It is prepared by gently heating butter until a clear golden liquid is obtained and a layer of milk solids coagulate at the bottom of the pan. The golden liquid is then carefully removed and cooled to form ghee. As most of the water content of the ghee has evaporated during the heating process, it is light, pure and resistant to spoilage. Unlike butter, ghee can be stored for years without refrigeration when kept in airtight containers.

According to Ayurvedic practice, ghee stimulates the secretion of stomach acids required for proper digestion. Many healers often prescribe ghee mixed with warm milk as a tonic for constipation. Ghee is also believed to help treat ulcers and colon inflammation, soothe stomach-aches, and promote healthy eyes and skin.

In Indian healing traditions, ghee is considered more alkaline than other oils; its frequent use is said to give smoother skin and a youthful look. Considered one of the best cooking mediums as it does not smoke or burn, ghee also rejuvenates body tissues such as nerves, bones, muscles, skin and hair, and is especially good for improving memory. For internal treatments, it is best to take fresh ghee that is less than a year old; ghee that has been stored for more than a year is excellent for massage treatments and can be used as a base oil for making herbal ointments for burns and skin rash.

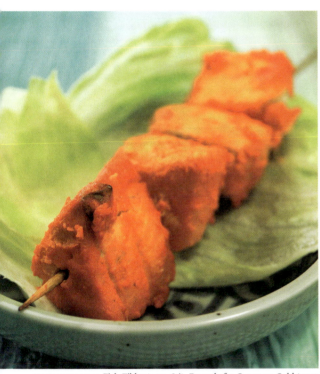 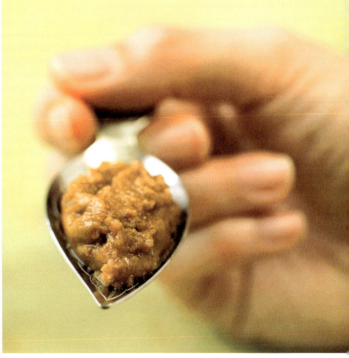

FROM LEFT TO RIGHT: *Fish Tikka (page 94), Remedy for Common Cold (page 93)*

Remedy for Common Cold

You can also take this remedy if you are suffering from indigestion or poor metabolism.

Ghee (clarified butter) 2 tsp
Ground ginger 2 tsp
Grated jaggery 2 tsp

Mix all ingredients together into a paste and take it first thing in the morning.

Take this remedy every morning until symptoms subside.

Fish Tikka

Preparation time: 15 minutes
Cooking time: 20 minutes
Serves: 6

Thick fish fillet 500 g (1 lb 1½ oz)
  cut into 2.5-cm (1-in) pieces

Natural yoghurt 200 ml
  (6⅔ fl oz / ¾ cup)

Chilli powder 1 tsp

Garam masala 1 tsp

Ginger paste 2 Tbsp

Garlic paste 2 Tbsp

Ajwain seeds 1 tsp

Chickpea flour (*besan*) 3 Tbsp

Salt 1½ tsp

Bright orange colouring a few drops

Melted ghee (clarified butter)
  for brushing

Wooden skewers

Put all ingredients except ghee into a mixing bowl and coat fish well. Set aside to marinate for 2 hours.

Skewer 4–5 marinated fish pieces onto a wooden skewer. Repeat until all fish pieces are used up.

Stand a metal rack on a baking tray and place skewered fish onto rack. Roast in a preheated oven at 180°C (350°F) for 10 minutes.

Remove and baste with ghee, then return to oven to roast for another 10 minutes, or until fish is cooked. Serve hot, on a bed of lettuce, if desired, with rice and other dishes.

Alu Paratha

Preparation time: 40 minutes
Cooking time: 10 minutes
Serves: 5

Potato Mixture

Potatoes 500 g (1 lb 1½ oz),
  boiled, peeled and mashed

Green chillies 2, finely chopped

Ginger 2-cm (1-in) knob, peeled and
  finely minced

Chopped coriander (cilantro)
  leaves 3 Tbsp

Turmeric powder ½ tsp

Salt 1 tsp

Dough

Fine wholemeal flour (atta flour)
  500 g (1lb 1½ oz) + extra for dusting

Salt 1¼ tsp

Lukewarm water 400 ml
  (13⅓ fl oz / 1⅝ cups)

Melted ghee (clarified butter)
  1½ Tbsp + extra for brushing

Place all ingredients for potato mixture into a bowl and combine well. Set aside.

Prepare dough. Combine all ingredients except ghee in a mixing bowl and knead to form a medium-soft dough. Add a little more water or flour, if dough is too dry or wet, respectively.

Knead dough well, about 8 minutes, then cover with cling film (plastic wrap) and set aside for 30 minutes.

Divide rested dough into balls about 5 cm (2-in) in diameter. Dust work surface with a little flour, then roll out each ball into a flat round and top with 2–3 Tbsp potato mixture. Bring dough up to enclose potato mixture inside and roll back into balls.

Roll out each potato-filled ball into a round paratha about 10 cm (4-in) in diameter.

Heat a frying pan (skillet) until hot, place a paratha on it and cook for about 1 minute. Turn paratha over and cook for another minute, brushing cooked side with a little melted ghee.

Turn paratha over again and cook greased side until golden brown and slightly crisp. Brush melted ghee on top, then turn over once more and cook until equally brown and crisp.

Remove to a flat plate and repeat until all paratha are cooked. Serve hot with a vegetable dish or curry.

Alu Paratha (page 94)

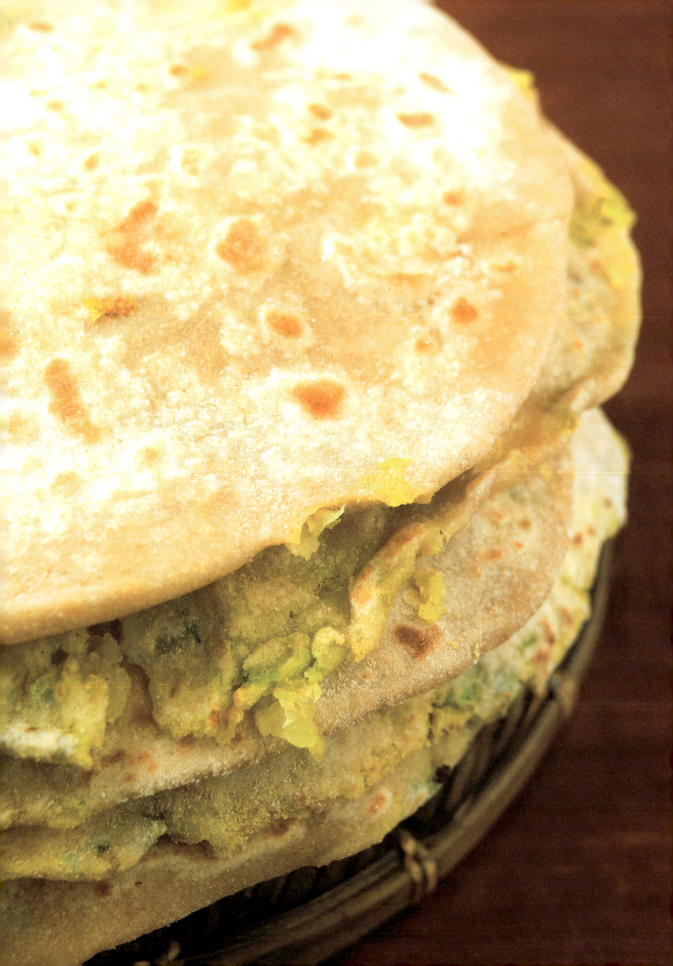

Ginger

Common Ginger, Common ginger, Stem ginger
Sanskrit Adraka (fresh), Sunthi (dried), Vishvabheshaja, Nagara
Tamil Inji, Ingee, Ingi, Shukku
Botanical Zingiber officinale

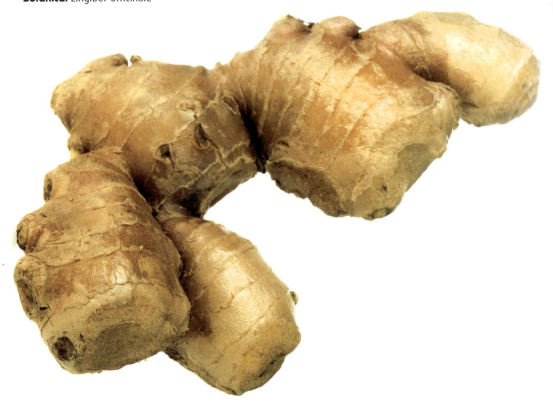

The fleshy, knobby stem or rhizome of the perennial ginger plant is used as a spice and to add a spicy, pungent kick to many dishes. Ginger is widely used in Indian cuisines as well as making pickles, curry powders and pastes. There are also many Indian sweet confections which are made with ginger.

In Indian cooking, the extremely hot juice extracted from 'old ginger' stems is often added to dishes to mask the strong flavours of seafood. A lot of ginger is also used in many Indian poultry and meat dishes, as ginger contains compounds similar to digestive enzymes which help ease the digestion of a heavy, protein-rich meal.

Dried powdered ginger is used to add a touch of spiciness to Indian desserts and sweets. As ginger powder lacks the pungency of fresh ginger and imparts a sweetish flavour to foods, the powder and fresh stem should not be substituted for each other.

Ginger is highly effective as a digestive aid and a carminative. By increasing the production of digestive fluids and saliva, ginger helps relieve flatulence, indigestion diarrhoea as well as stomach cramps. It is also used in natural remedies to alleviate nausea caused by motion or morning sickness.

Possessing anti-inflammatory properties, ginger is also effective in easing the pain and reducing the inflammation of arthritic or rheumatic joints. The spice is also taken to warm the body in order to promote perspiration which helps to detoxify the system and put a stop to persistent fevers. High blood pressure may be lowered with the use of ginger. The spice is also an expectorant, useful in loosening and expelling phlegm from the lungs when one suffers from bronchitis or asthma.

In recent times, ginger tea has been recommended to alleviate nausea in patients undergoing chemotherapy as its natural properties do not interact in a negative way with other medications. However, it is important to discuss the medicinal use of ginger with a physician before taking it as excess use can lead to gastric irritation.

Ginger Compress

This compress helps to stimulate blood circulation and is especially helpful for those who suffer from painful rheumatic joints.

Ginger 150 g (5¹/₃ oz), peeled and grated

Hot water (not boiling) 2 litres (64 fl oz / 8 cups)

Place grated ginger into a small muslin bag and secure.

Squeeze ginger juice from muslin bag into a basin of hot water, then immerse bag in the basin and leave for about 5 minutes.

Dip a clean cotton towel into liquid and wring cloth dry. Apply hot towel to affected part of the body.

Using another thick dry towel, cover the damp towel to keep the heat in for a while. Replace the damp towel with a hot one every 3 minutes, or until the skin becomes slightly flushed.

Ginger Sesame Massage Oil

This oil relieves general aches and also helps in improving blood circulation.

Ginger juice 3 Tbsp
Gingelly oil 3 Tbsp

Whisk ingredients together with a fork briskly for 1 minute, until an emulsion is formed.

Use prepared oil to gently massage the aching parts of the body.

Cough Remedy

Indian long pepper 1 tsp

Ginger powder 1 tsp

Holy basil leaf powder 1 tsp

Cardamoms 10

Honey

Grind all ingredients except honey together into a fine powder. Store in an airtight container for use as required.

Whenever you feel yourself developing a cough, mix 1 tsp prepared powder with 1 tsp honey to a paste. Suck on paste and allow it to slowly dissolve in the mouth.

Ginger and Mango Chutney

Preparation time: 15 minutes
Cooking time: 25 minutes
Serves: 8

Unripe mangoes 5, medium, peeled, stoned and diced

Ginger 120 g (4^1/$_2$ oz), peeled and julienned

Chilli powder 1^1/$_2$ tsp

Raisins or chopped seedless dates 250 g (9 oz)

Cinnamon powder ^{1}/$_2$ tsp

Cardamom powder ^{1}/$_2$ tsp

Grated jaggery 500 g (1 lb 1^1/$_2$ oz)

White vinegar 300 ml (10 fl oz/1^1/$_4$ cups)

Salt ^{1}/$_2$ tsp

Place all ingredients into a heavy-based saucepan.

Stir occasionally and cook over low heat for 20 minutes or until chutney is thick and mangoes turn pulpy.

Cool thoroughly before storing in sterilised glass jars.

Refrigerate for at least 3 days before serving. Chutney can be stored, refrigerated, for up to a year.

Ginger Tuvayal

This dish promotes digestion and therefore is perfect for accompanying a large meal.

Preparation time: 10 minutes
Cooking time: 10 minutes
Serves: 6

Cooking oil 2 tsp

Skinned split black lentils (*urad* dhal) 2 tsp

Coriander seeds 2 Tbsp

Dried chillies 12, cut into smaller pieces

Ginger 300 g (10^1/$_2$ oz), peeled and cut into small pieces

Curry leaves 3 sprigs, stems discarded

Tamarind pulp 100 g (3^1/$_2$ oz), mixed with 150 ml (5 fl oz / ^{5}/$_8$ cup) water and strained

Asafoetida powder ^{1}/$_2$ tsp

Grated jaggery 2 Tbsp

Salt 1^1/$_4$ tsp

Heat oil and fry lentils until golden brown. Drain and remove to a plate.

In same oil, add coriander seeds, dried chillies, ginger and curry leaves and sauté over low heat until aromatic, about 3 minutes.

Transfer to a blender (processor), add all remaining ingredients and blend (process) to obtain a smooth texture. Serve with rice and other dishes.

CLOCKWISE FROM TOP: Ginger and Mango Chutney (page 98), Ginger Tuvayal (page 98), Cough Remedy (page 98)

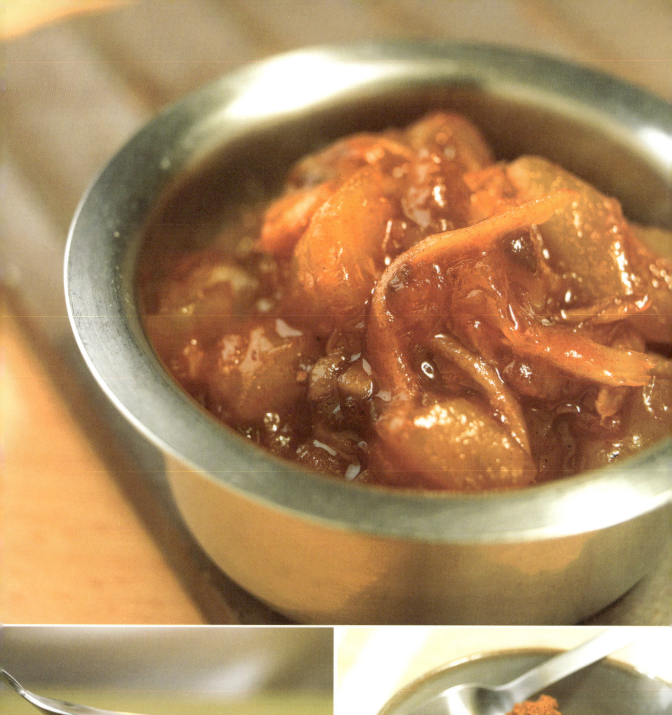

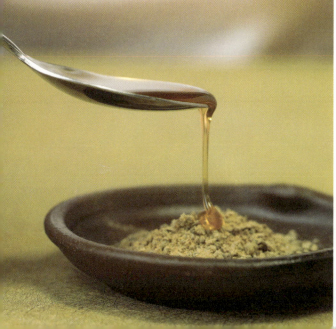

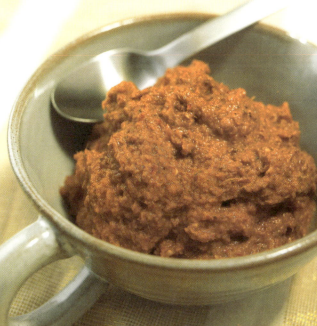

Henna

Henna is a green plant which looks similar to a tea shrub and has been known for centuries for its excellent hair conditioning, dyeing and colouring properties. Henna powder is a preparation made purely from ground dried henna leaves.

In India, many women apply henna designs to beautify themselves for special occasions such as weddings and religious holidays. Hindus associate henna closely with Lakshmi, the Hindu goddess of wealth and fortune. As henna contains cooling and antibacterial properties, the powder is often applied in poultices to treat external burns and bruises. Henna poultices can also help lower the body temperature to soothe fevers and headaches. Used as a natural hair conditioner and dye, henna regulates the secretion of scalp oil to provide a healthy lustre to the hair. It is an excellent remedy for almost all scalp disorders including dandruff and hair loss.

Common Henna
Sanskrit Mendika, Ragangi
Tamil Marudaani
Botanical Lawsonia Inermis

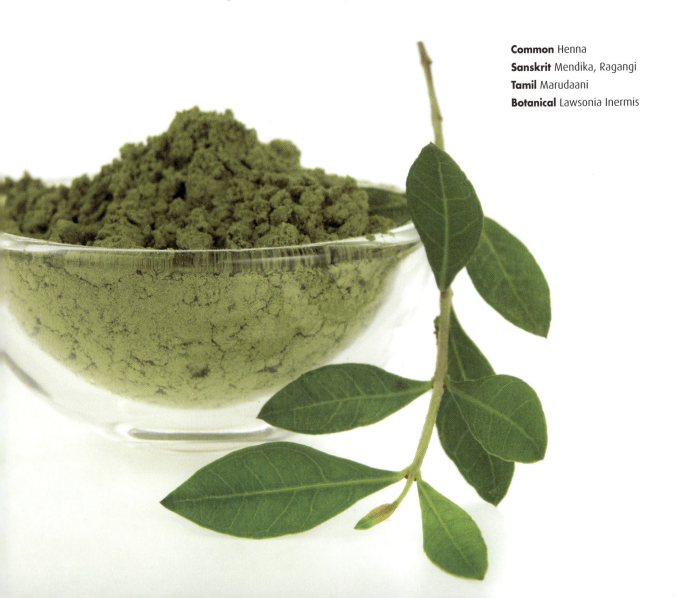

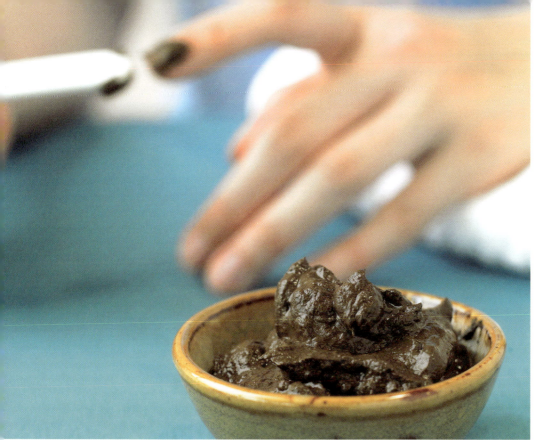

Nail Conditioner (page 101)

Nail Conditioner

Remove existing nail polish a day or two before treatment. Remember to stir the paste each time before you apply onto your nails.

Warm distilled water
  50 ml (1²/₃ fl oz / ¹/₄ cup)

Henna powder 1 heaped Tbsp

Natural yoghurt 2 Tbsp

Eucalyptus oil 2-3 drops

In a stainless steel or porcelain bowl, mix all ingredients to form a paste.

To avoid hands from getting stained, cut 1 cm off the fingertips of disposable gloves before wearing them. Using an applicator, apply tiny globes of henna paste onto each exposed, clean and dry nail and cuticle. Make sure each fingernail is well-covered.

Leave on for 10 minutes. If you have time, put both hands into a clean plastic bag and cover with a towel for up to ¹/₂ hour.

Rinse fingers with lukewarm water and towel-dry.

Henna Hair Mask

Apply this mask once a month and see your crowning glory grow shiny and healthy!

Henna powder 250 g (9 oz)

Indian gooseberry powder 2 tsp

Lemon juice 4 Tbsp

Coffee powder 2 tsp

Black tea leaves 2 tsp

Natural yoghurt 150 ml (5 fl oz / ⁵/₈ cup)

Gingelly oil 1 tsp

Egg 1, medium, lightly beaten

Combine all ingredients except egg in a stainless steel or porcelain bowl.

Set aside for about 12 hours. Stir egg into mixture and apply onto hair, then comb through hair with a wide-tooth comb to ensure even and thorough application.

Leave on for 1 hour, then rinse off and shampoo hair as usual.

Hibiscus

Common Hibiscus, Shoe-flower
Sanskrit Rogapushpa, Japapushpa
Tamil Semparuthi
Botanical Hibiscus rosa-sinensis

The hibiscus flower is known for its beauty as well as its herbal applications. The edible flower can be added to salads for colour and is also used in jams and jellies to impart a tart, refreshing taste. In Indian cuisine, the petals are dipped in a light batter and deep-fried into a light, crispy fritter known as Bhaji.

As hibiscus flowers contain citric acid, they are used as a cooling herb for making refreshing drinks to provide relief during the hot weather. The leaves and roots of the hibiscus plant are used in various folk remedies. Hibiscus tea made from hibiscus flowers has a mild laxative effect on the body and is also effective in dissolving phlegm in the system caused by coughs and colds. Red hibiscus flowers are especially high in vitamin C content.

The hibiscus flower is also known to contain components that lower the blood pressure. A natural emollient, the leaves and flowers of the hibiscus plant are used all over the world for softening or healing the skin and as a natural hair conditioner. Leaves are warmed and placed on cracked feet or on boils and ulcers to promote healing while petals are used in recipes for conditioning the hair.

Natural Hair Conditioner

This simple and natural conditioner is great for softening the hair.

Fresh hibiscus flowers 6 blooms
Water for soaking

Immerse hibiscus flowers in water for about 1 hour. Drain and reserve soaking water.

Grind hibiscus flowers with 100 ml (3^1/$_3$ fl oz / ^{3}/$_8$ cup) water into a paste.

Use ground paste like a shampoo to wash hair (the paste has a soapy texture).

Rinse hair with water and use soaking water set aside earlier for a final rinse.

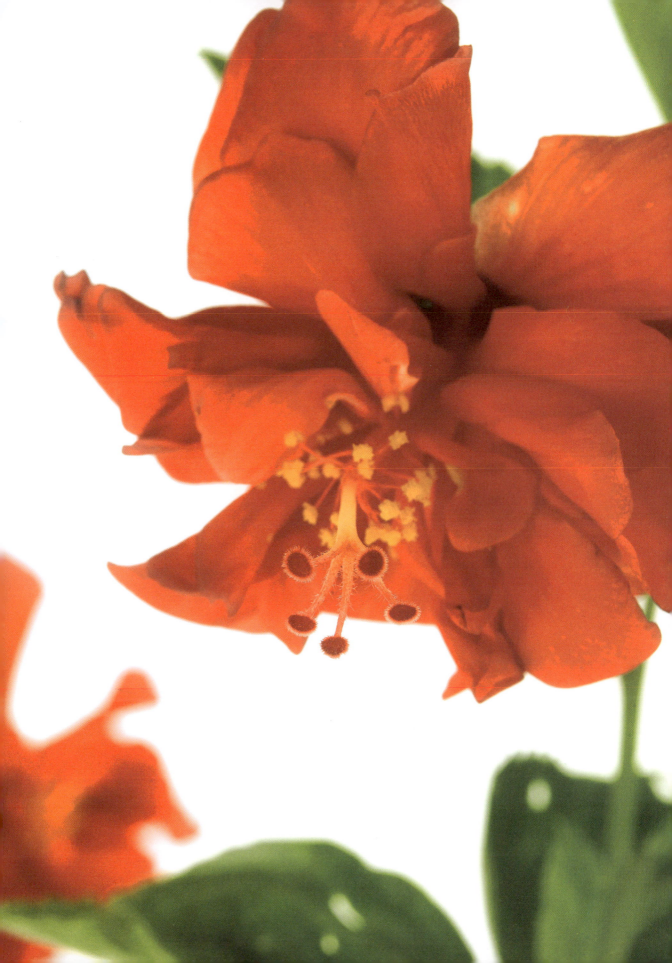

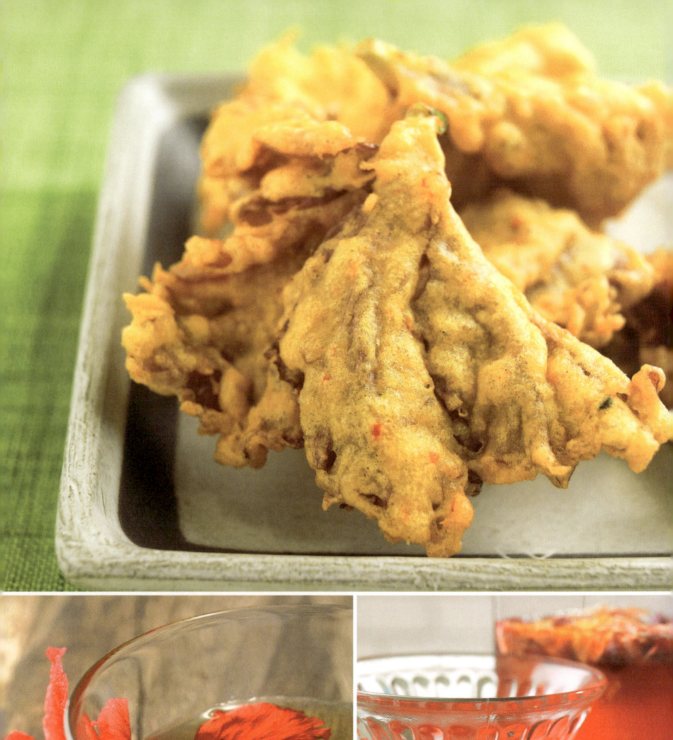

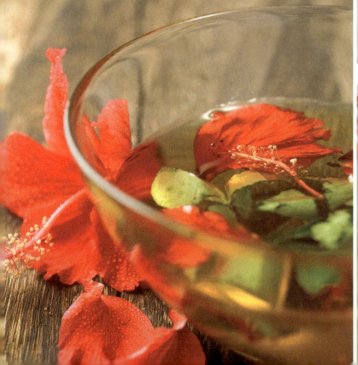

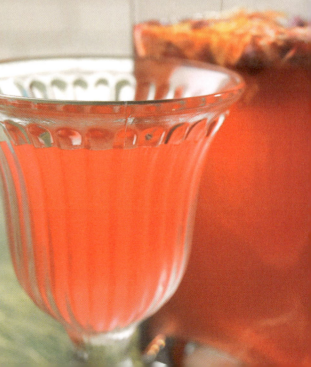

Hibiscus Hair Tonic

Massage this oil onto the scalp and hair and leave on for about 1 hour before shampooing. It helps to arrest premature greying and also maintain the natural pigment of the hair. Your hair will become silky soft too.

Hibiscus powder or dried hibiscus flowers 50 g (2 oz)

Dried jasmine leaves 30 g (1 oz)

Gingelly oil 400 ml (13$^1/_3$ fl oz / 1$^5/_8$ cups)

Rose or lavender essential oil 4 drops

Place hibiscus powder or flowers and jasmine leaves into a clean, dry glass bottle. Set aside.

Warm gingelly oil slightly. Add essential oil and stir well. When completely cool, add to bottle with hibiscus and jasmine leaves.

Leave oil aside in a dark place at room temperature for one month before using.

Note: The oil can be stored for up to 5–6 months.

Hibiscus Syrup

Fresh red hibiscus flowers 300 g (10$^1/_2$ oz)

Lime juice 100 ml (3$^1/_3$ fl oz / $^3/_8$ cup)

Sugar 400 g (14 oz)

Water 500 ml (16 fl oz / 2 cups)

Soak hibiscus flowers in water for 10 minutes to remove any trace of pesticide, then rinse before use. Soak hibiscus flowers in lime juice for 20 minutes.

Put sugar and water in a pot and bring to the boil for 10 minutes.

Add flowers and lime juice mixture. Boil until almost reduced by half and mixture turns syrupy.

Strain and when cool, store syrup in a clean and dry glass bottle. Serve as a refreshing drink, mixed with iced water.

Hibiscus Bhaji

Hibiscus flowers 10 blooms

Water 450 ml (14 fl oz / 1$^3/_4$ cups)

Chickpea flour (besan) 300 g (10$^1/_2$ oz), sifted

Garlic paste 2 Tbsp

Ginger paste 1 Tbsp

Rice flour 2 Tbsp, sifted

Turmeric powder 1 tsp

Curry powder 1 tsp

Baking powder $^1/_2$ tsp

Salt 1 tsp

Cumin seeds $^1/_2$ tsp

Cooking oil for deep-frying

Separate petals of hibiscus flowers, discarding stamens and sepals. Soak in water for 10 minutes to remove any trace of pesticide. Drain, then rinse and pat dry thoroughly on absorbent paper towels. Set aside.

Put remaining ingredients except cooking oil into a deep mixing bowl and mix well to form a smooth batter. Set aside for 15 minutes.

Dip hibiscus petals into prepared batter and deep-fry in hot oil until golden brown. Drain on absorbent paper towels and serve hot as a snack.

Holy Basil

Holy basil is a sturdy and very aromatic herb with a minty-grassy scent and pale green leafy stems covered with very fine hairs. This herb has great religious and medicinal significance in India since the Vedic times; the plant is sacred to Lord Vishnu, the Hindu god of preservation and is regarded as cleansing for the body, mind and spirit. Believed to provide divine protection for the home, holy basil is grown by many Hindus in the home for use in religious worship. As a medicinal herb, holy basil leaves are used to brew a strong tea for the treatment of flu. It is also soothing for the stomach; fresh or powdered dried leaves taken after meals will help ease indigestion. Recent research has also confirmed that holy basil aids in stabilising blood sugar levels, lowering blood pressure and relieving stress. For external treatments, the juice of fresh leaves, which has antibiotic qualities can be applied topically to skin conditions including acne and allergic rash.

Common Holy basil
Sanskrit Ajaka, Arjaka. Brinda Gauri, Tulsi
Tamil Alungai, Karut tulasi, Kullai, Tulasi, Nalla thulasi
Botanical Ocimum tenuiflorum

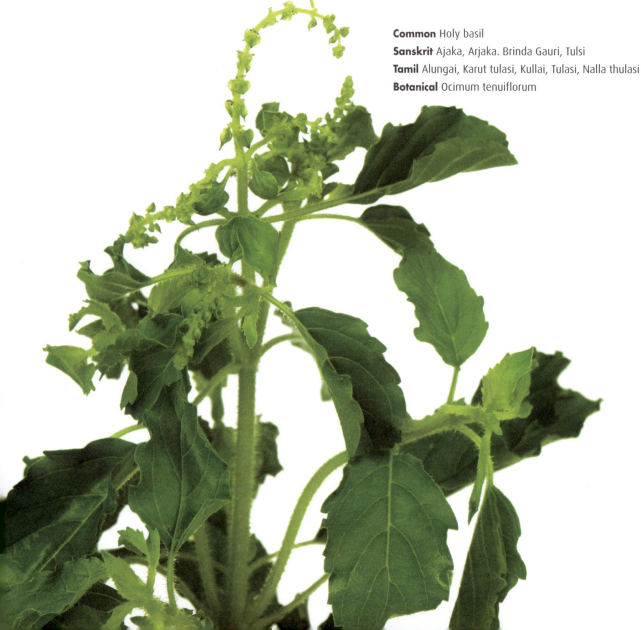

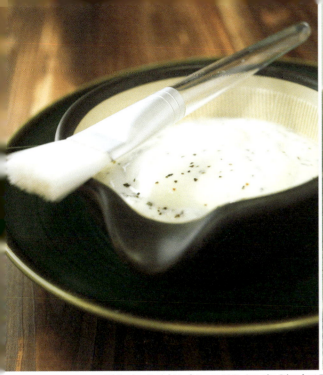
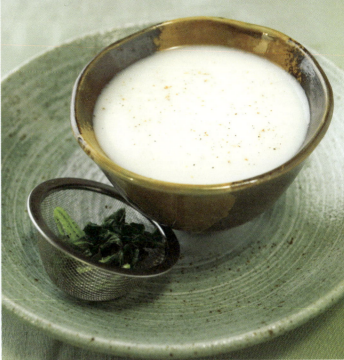

FROM LEFT TO RIGHT: Whitening Facial Mask (page 107), Appetite Stimulant Tea (page 107)

Whitening Facial Mask

With regular use, this mask will remove light spots such as freckles on the skin.

Dried holy basil leaf powder 2 Tbsp
Yoghurt 2 Tbsp

Mix all ingredients together into a paste and apply on the face and neck.

Leave on for 30 minutes. Rinse off and pat dry with a clean towel.

Appetite Stimulant Tea

The holy basil plant has appetite-enhancing properties; drinking this tea will help to enhance your appetite.

Holy basil leaves 40 g (1¹/₂ oz)
Water 300 ml (10 fl oz / 1¹/₄ cups)
Hot fresh milk 250 ml (8 fl oz / 1 cup)
Cardamoms 2, pounded
Sugar to taste

Boil basil leaves in water until liquid is reduced by half.

Strain tea and add milk. Add pounded cardamoms and stir in sugar to taste. Serve hot. This tea can be drunk up to twice a day.

General Body-wellness Remedy

For general well-being, chew this concoction twice a day for stress relief. Basil leaves also help purify the blood and prevent the onset of many common ailments such as coughs and colds.

Holy basil leaves 10
Black peppercorns 2, crushed

Mix all ingredients together, then chew for 10 minutes and discard.

Repeat twice a day to keep well.

Honey

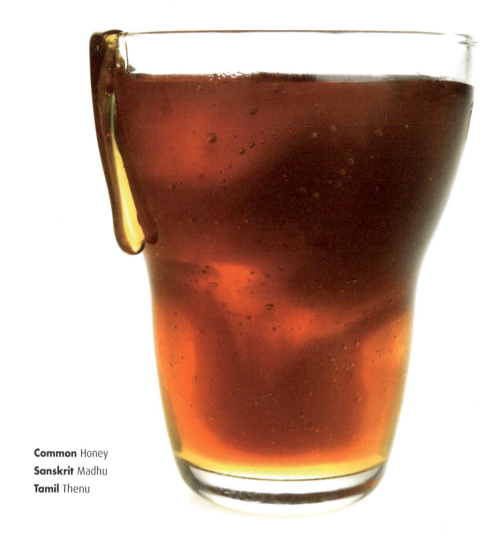

Common Honey
Sanskrit Madhu
Tamil Thenu

An essential ingredient in the stock cupboards of many Indian homes, honey is used for religious purposes, food and medicine as well as beauty treatments. The consistency of honey ranges from rather viscous to very thin; in colour from dark to nearly clear.

It is believed that honey is easily assimilated by the body and gentle on the digestive system. In traditional Indian healing, honey is added to many herbal preparations as it does not alter the chemical balance of remedies and helps transport the medicine directly into the blood stream, enabling these preparations to be more effectively absorbed by the body. With a sweet and astringent taste, honey is highly effective in removing phelgm from the system. It helps to soothe the inflamed mucous membrane of the upper respiratory tract as well as provide relief for persistent coughs. A mixture of one teaspoon of honey with an equal proportion of ginger juice in a single dose, is used by many Indian grandmothers to treat their grandchildren when they are down with coughs and runny noses. A gargle of honey mixed with water also provides relief for sore throats. For those suffering from high blood pressure, a daily dose of two teaspoons of honey mixed with one teaspoon of garlic juice is believed to be beneficial.

Some older Indians drink a glass of warm water mixed with the juice of half a lemon daily before breakfast as it is purported to be an effective cure for constipation and hyperacidity. Honey contains antioxidant properties which render it useful in external treatments; it helps to restore damaged skin and keep the skin youthful and supple. Honey is a common ingredient in moisturisers, masks and other beauty treatments as it has natural hydrating properties. Possessing antioxidant qualities, honey also has the ability to protect the skin from damage caused by the sun's UV rays.

Honey Rejuvenating Mask

Use this hydrating mask frequently to keep your skin smooth and wrinkle-free.

Honey 3 Tbsp

White sesame seeds 2 Tbsp, coarsely pounded

Mix all ingredients together and apply a thin layer on clean face, avoiding the eye contours.

Leave on for at least 30 minutes, then rinse off thoroughly with tepid water and pat dry with a clean towel.

FROM LEFT TO RIGHT: *Honey Rejuvenating Mask (page 109), Parsi Roast Chicken (page 110)*

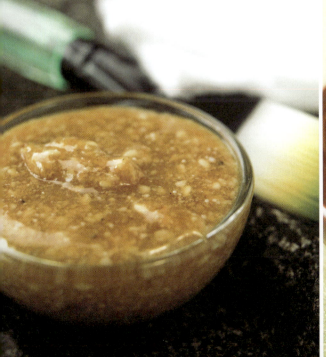
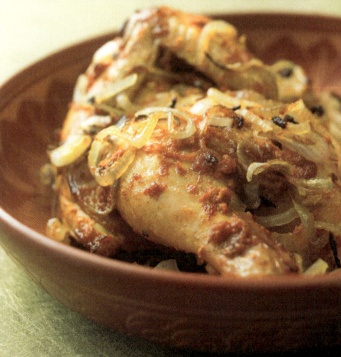

Stuffed Pea Cutlets

Preparation time: 15 minutes
Cooking time: 15 minutes
Serves: 6

Frozen peas 500 g (1 lb 1^1/$_2$ oz), thawed

Rice flour 140 g (5 oz)

Honey 2 Tbsp

Lemon juice 1 Tbsp

Grated coconut 30 g (1 oz)

Cashew nuts 80 g (3 oz), finely chopped

Green chillies 4, finely chopped

Garam masala 1^1/$_2$ tsp

Cooking oil for deep-frying

Blend (process) peas in a blender (processor) until a coarse paste is formed. Transfer to a mixing bowl.

Add all remaining ingredients to mixing bowl except cooking oil. Combine well and shape mixture into patties, 3 cm (1.5-in) in diameter.

Deep-fry patties until lightly browned. Drain on absorbent paper towels and serve hot as a snack.

Pimple Treatment

Apply this paste on the pimples before bedtime and rinse off the next morning with warm water. Repeat this treatment daily for two weeks for best results.

Honey 1 Tbsp

Cinnamon powder 1 tsp

Mix all ingredients together and dab onto pimples before bedtime.

Rinse off thoroughly the next morning and pat dry with a clean towel.

Parsi Roast Chicken

Preparation time: 4 hours
Cooking time: 40 minutes
Serves: 6

Chicken 1, halved

Onions 2, large, peeled and cut into rings

Marinade

Red chillies 8, stalks discarded and left whole

Garlic 5 cloves, peeled and left whole

Ginger 3-cm (1^1/$_2$-in) knob, peeled

Onion 1, medium, peeled and quartered

Fennel seeds 1^1/$_2$ tsp

Garam masala 1^1/$_2$ tsp

Turmeric powder 1 tsp

Ghee (clarified butter) 1 tsp

Finely chopped coriander (cilantro) leaves 3 Tbsp

Honey 2 Tbsp

Salt 1^1/$_2$ tsp

Blend (process) ingredients for marinade in a blender (processor) until smooth.

Rub marinade all over chicken and set aside for 4 hours.

Arrange onion rings on top of marinated chicken and roast on the middle rack of a preheated oven at 180°C (350°F) for 35 minutes, or until chicken is cooked through and golden brown. Serve hot with rice and other dishes.

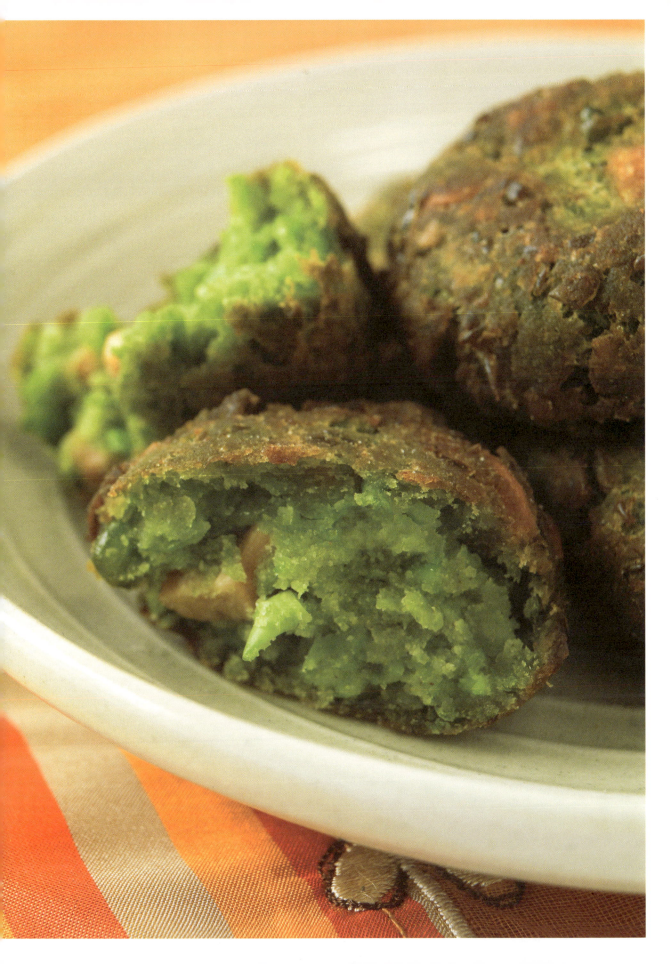

Indian Gooseberry

Common Indian gooseberry, Emblic myrobalan
Sanskrit Amalaki, Dhatriphala
Tamil Nelli, Nellkai, Amalakam, Ambal, Amla
Botanical Phyllanthus emblica

The Indian gooseberry is an amazing fruit which can be described as one of the most precious gifts of nature to mankind. It is one of the richest known natural sources of vitamin C and regarded as the best herbal medicine for rejuvenation in Ayurveda. A sacred tree that is symbolic of Mother Earth in India for the nourishing fruits it bears, it is commonly grown in the compounds of homes and Hindu temples.

In Indian cooking, the fresh fruits are often used for making pickles and preserves. The extremely tangy fruit has many medicinal properties and is used as a diuretic as well as a laxative. The astringent fruit is also believed to be capable of slowing down the ageing process and strengthening the body's resistance against infectious diseases. Other traditional applications of the Indian gooseberry fruit include, in the treatment of skin diseases, indigestion and lung problems.

Dried Indian gooseberry fruits are also used in Ayurvedic medicine for treating fever, liver disorder, anaemia and urinary tract conditions. One remedy prescribes a mixture of bittergourd juice and Indian gooseberry juice to be drunk for regulating the blood sugar level in the treatment of diabetes. Modern research has also shown that Indian gooseberries are effective in lowering the blood cholesterol levels and therefore useful in the treatment of heart disease.

For the treatment of rheumatism, one teaspoonful of the dried fruit powder may be mixed with two teaspoonfuls of jaggery in a single dose, to be taken twice daily for up to a month. For external applications, the Indian gooseberry is traditionally regarded as an excellent hair tonic, useful in promoting hair growth and preventing the premature greying of hair.

Hair Mask

This is a great treatment for attaining soft and silky hair and also for stimulating hair growth.

Ground dried Indian gooseberries 100 g (3^1/$_3$ oz)
Henna powder 100 g (3^1/$_3$ oz)
Water 100 ml (3^1/$_3$ fl oz / ^{3}/$_8$ cup)

Put all ingredients into a stainless steel or porcelain bowl and stir to mix well. Set aside for 20 minutes.

Massage into hair and scalp. Leave on for 30 minutes. Rinse off and shampoo hair as usual.

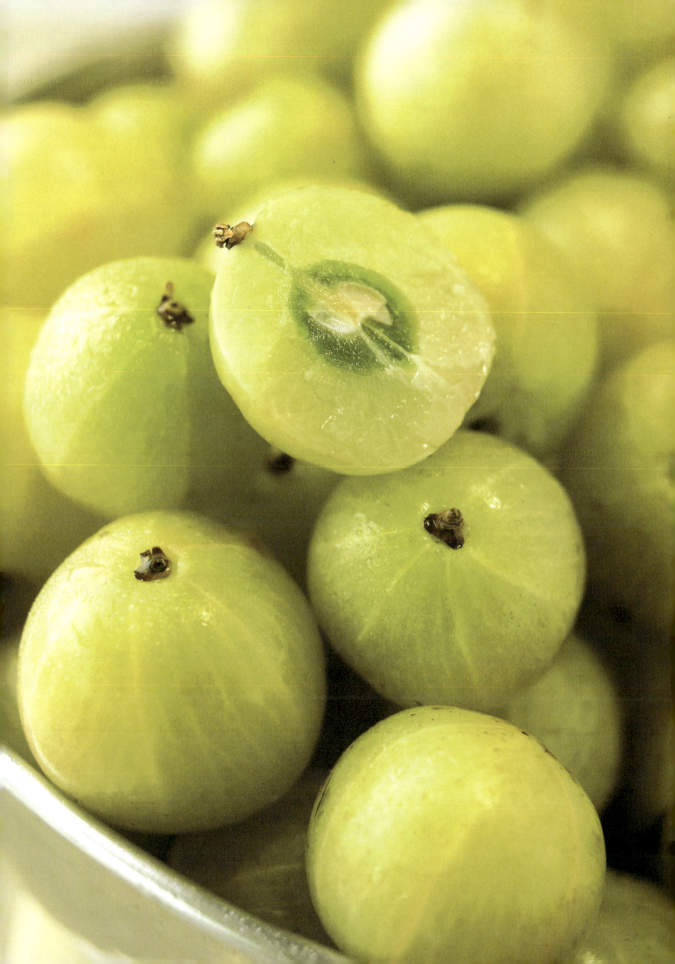

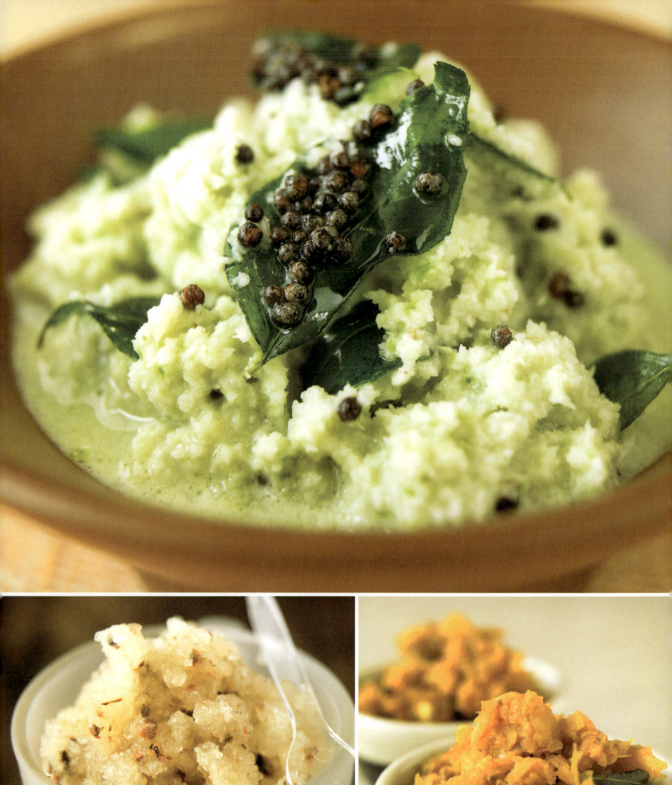
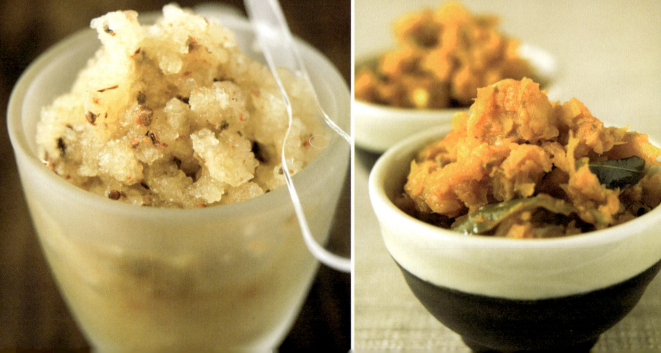

Nellkai Chammandhi

Preparation time: 15 minutes
Cooking time: 3 minutes
Serves: 6

Ripe Indian gooseberries 10

Green chillies 5, cut into 1-cm (^{1}/$_2$-in) pieces

Ginger 2-cm (1-in) knob, peeled

Shallots 100 g (3^1/$_2$ oz), peeled and left whole

Salt 1 tsp

Grated coconut 100 g (3 ^{1}/$_2$ oz)

Gingelly oil 1 Tbsp

Black mustard seeds 1 tsp

Curry leaves 2 sprigs, stems discarded

Halve gooseberries and remove seeds.

Blend gooseberries, chillies, ginger, shallots, salt and coconut together in a blender (processor) until smooth. Transfer to a serving bowl.

Heat oil in a separate pan and fry mustard seeds until they stop spluttering. Add curry leaves and sauté for a few seconds.

Remove from heat and add sautéed mixture to serving bowl. Stir to combine well and serve with thosai or rice.

Appetite Stimulant

Cloves 4

Nutmeg 1

Indian long pepper 2

Ginger powder ^{1}/$_2$ tsp

Indian gooseberries 15

Caster (superfine) sugar 1 Tbsp

Grind all ingredients together in a spice grinder into a paste.

Consume this portion twice a day to regain lost appetite due to illness.

Amla Thokku

Preparation time: 20 minutes
Cooking time: 5 minutes
Serves: 8

Indian gooseberries 600 g (1 lb 5 oz)

Gingelly oil 300 ml (10 fl oz / 1^1/$_4$ cups)

Black mustard seeds 1^1/$_2$ tsp

Asafoetida powder 1^1/$_2$ tsp

Ginger 450 g (1 lb), peeled and coarsely chopped

Green chillies 200 g (7 oz), coarsely chopped

Curry leaves 5 sprigs, stems discarded

Tamarind pulp 200 g (7 oz), mixed with 200 ml (6^2/$_3$ fl oz / ^{3}/$_4$ cup) water and strained

Chilli powder 20 g (^{2}/$_3$ oz)

Sugar 2 tsp

Fenugreek seeds 20 g (^{2}/$_3$ oz), coarsely ground

Salt 3 tsp

Rice vinegar 100 ml (3^1/$_3$ fl oz / ^{3}/$_8$ cup)

Pound gooseberries coarsely and remove seeds.

Heat oil until foaming, then add mustards seeds and stir-fry until they stop spluttering.

Add asafoetida powder, ginger, green chillies and curry leaves and sauté for 2 minutes.

Add remaining ingredients together with pounded gooseberries.

Bring to the boil and remove from heat immediately. Leave to cool completely before storing in clean, airtight glass jars.

Refrigerate for up to a week before serving as a condiment with rice or bread.

Note: The condiment can refrigerate well for up to half a year.

Indian Long Pepper

Common Indian long pepper
Sanskrit Pippali, Magandhi, Kana, Ushana
Tamil Kandan lippilli, Pippili, Sirumulam, Tippili
Botanical Piper longum

For centuries, the Indian long pepper has been used as a herbal spice and medicine in India. Long and cylindrical, the long pepper has a warm, musky aroma with slightly sweet overtones. Since long pepper is more pungent than black pepper, use it in small quantities to flavour the food when cooking. Crush the pepper rods before use to fully release their aroma. In India, long peppers are often used in pickles or spicy, clear soups.

In traditional Indian healing, long peppers are most commonly used in remedies for treating respiratory ailments such as coughs and bronchitis. The spice is also used in the treatment of stomach disorders, diseases of the spleen, tumours and asthma. Long pepper is applied in remedies for relieving muscular pains and inflammation. Containing antibacterial properties, long pepper is often introduced to young Indian children in medicinal soups for building up their immunity against many infections.

Cough Remedy

Indian long pepper powder $^1/_2$ tsp
Turmeric powder $1^1/_2$ tsp
Ajwain powder 1 tsp
Honey 1 tsp

Mix all ingredients together to combine well and consume this portion twice a day (in the morning and evening) until cough subsides.

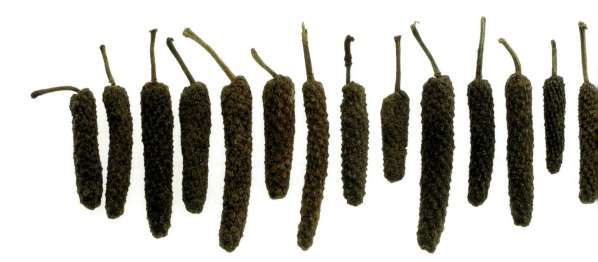

Long Pepper Mutton

Preparation time: 4 hours
Cooking time: 60 minutes
Serves: 5

Boneless mutton 1 kg (2 lb 3 oz), cut into large cubes

Garlic 6 cloves, peeled and left whole

Ginger 3-cm (1 1/2-in) knob, peeled and sliced

Chilli powder 2 Tbsp

Coriander (cilantro) powder 2 Tbsp

Turmeric powder 1 tsp

Salt 1/2 tsp

Curry leaves 1 sprig, stem discarded

Water 1 litre (32 fl oz / 4 cups)

Spice Mixture

Cooking oil 3 Tbsp

Black mustard seeds 1 tsp

Shallots or onions 150 g (5 1/3 oz), peeled and sliced

Green chillies 5, slit lengthwise

Ginger 2-cm (1-in) knob, peeled and julienned

Curry leaves 2 sprigs, stems discarded

Indian long peppers 4, coarsely pounded

Black peppercorns 1 tsp, coarsely pounded

Garam masala 1 1/2 tsp

Place all ingredients except spice mixture into a pot and boil over medium heat until meat is almost tender.

Prepare spice mixture. Heat oil in a wok, then add mustard seeds and stir-fry until they stop spluttering.

Add shallots or onions, chillies, ginger and curry leaves and sauté until shallots or onions turn golden brown. Add long peppers and peppercorns, then sauté until aromatic. Finally, stir in garam masala.

Add spice mixture to mutton and cook, stirring occasionally over high heat until gravy has thickened and mutton is well-coated. Serve with rice or bread.

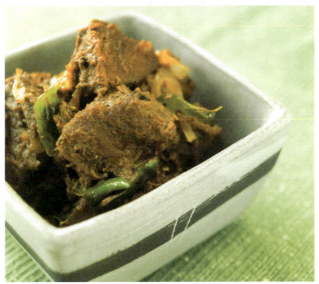

Long Pepper Mutton (page 117)

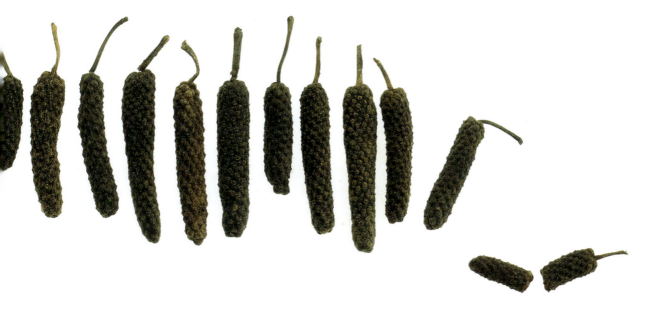

Indian Pennywort

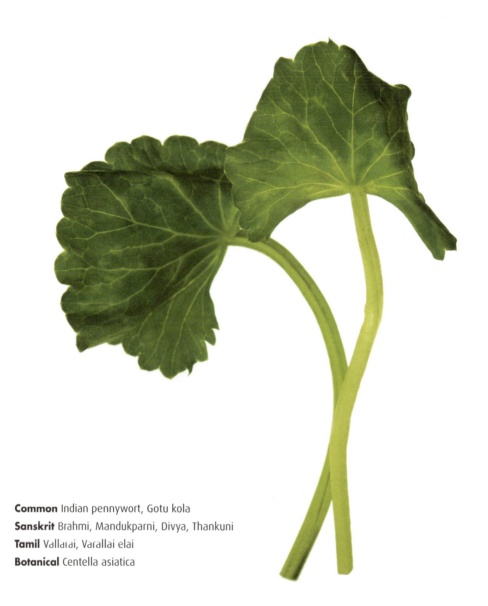

Common Indian pennywort, Gotu kola
Sanskrit Brahmi, Mandukparni, Divya, Thankuni
Tamil Vallarai, Varallai elai
Botanical Centella asiatica

Indian pennywort, also commonly known as gotu kola, is a perennial creeper that thrives in marshlands throughout India. The herb has small, fan-shaped green leaves and bears small white flowers. The fresh leaves of the Indian pennywort are widely used in Indian cooking and are served in soups, chutneys, salads, breads or even juiced.

The leaves and stems of the gotu kola plant are used for many medicinal treatments, including for skin diseases, stomach ailments and nervous disorders. In traditional Indian healing, the herb is a highly prized tonic for its efficacy in improving memory and mental clarity as well as its wound-healing properties. To effectively reduce anxiety and improve mental concentration, a combination of gotu kola and meditation practice is often prescribed. Some other Indian folk remedies include taking soups cooked with gotu kola to help chronic skin ulcers and other wounds heal better and faster.

For external treatments, fresh or dried gotu kola leaves and stems are also made into poultices and applied onto wounds or skin rash to aid healing. As the herb has a calming effect on both the mind and body, gotu kola is also useful in the treatment of insomnia and indigestion; a tea brewed with gotu kola leaves, sweetened with honey and taken before bedtime can help induce a restful sleep or relieve indigestion due to a poor diet or overeating.

Gotu Kola Sambol

Preparation time: 15 minutes
Serves: 4

Indian pennywort leaves 350 g (12^1/$_2$ oz), very finely shredded

Shallots 8, peeled and thinly sliced

Green chillies 2, sliced

Lime juice 3 Tbsp

Grated coconut 60 g (2 oz)

Salt 1 tsp

Combine all ingredients together and serve with rice and other dishes.

Tea for Indigestion

Indian pennywort leaves 30 g (1 oz)

Ginger powder 30 g (1 oz)

Garlic cloves 30 g (1 oz), peeled and pounded

Water 1 litre (32 fl oz / 4 cups)

Boil all ingredients together until liquid is reduced to about 250 ml (8 fl oz / 1 cup).

Drink often if suffering from indigestion.

FROM LEFT TO RIGHT: *Vallarai Porridge (page 120), Tea for Indigestion (page 119)*

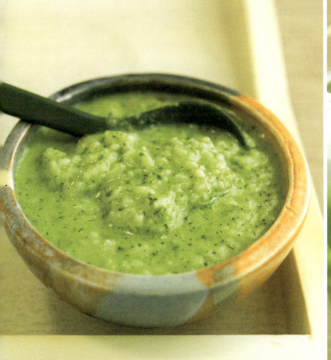
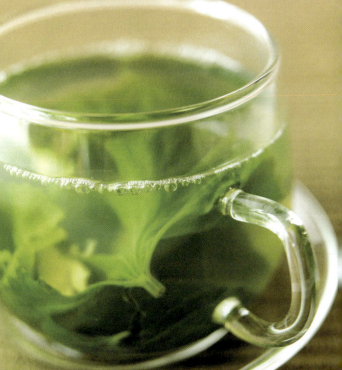

Gotu Kola Tea

Drinking this tea regularly helps to 'cool' the body as well as regulate the nervous and circulatory systems.

Indian pennywort leaves 10

Boiling water 250 ml (8 fl oz / 1 cup)

Honey 1 tsp

Put leaves into a mug and pour boiling water over.

Leave to steep until drink cools completely.

Stir in honey and drink.

Gotu Kola Sothi

Preparation time: 15 minutes
Cooking time: 10 minutes
Serves: 6

Cooking oil 2 Tbsp

Black mustard seeds 1 tsp

Cumin seeds 1 tsp

Fenugreek seeds $1/2$ tsp

Onion 1, peeled and sliced

Dried prawns (shrimps) 50 g (2 oz),
soaked, drained and pounded

Curry leaves 2 sprigs, stems discarded

Thin coconut milk 1 litre
(32 fl oz / 4 cups) (see page 50)

Turmeric powder $1/2$ tsp

Red chilli 1, cut into 1-cm
($1/2$-in) pieces

Indian pennywort leaves 250 g (9 oz)

Salt $1/2$ tsp

Thick coconut milk 250 ml
(8 fl oz / 1 cup) (see page 50)

Heat oil and fry mustard, cumin and fenugreek seeds until aromatic.

Add onion, dried prawns and curry leaves and fry until onion turns golden brown.

Add thin coconut milk, turmeric powder and chilli.

Boil for 3 minutes. Add Indian pennywort leaves, salt and thick coconut milk.

Bring to the boil, stirring constantly. Remove from heat and serve immediately with rice.

Vallarai Porridge

The Vallarai Porridge is a thick, nutritious mixture of broken rice grains, coconut milk and blended Indian pennywort leaves. It is a great breakfast dish that contains all the necessary carbohydrates, vitamins and minerals to kick-start the day with.

Broken rice grains 100 g (3$1/2$ oz),
washed and drained

Water 1 litre (32 fl oz / 4 cups)

Thick coconut milk 200 ml
(6 $2/3$ fl oz / $3/4$ cup) (see page 50)

Indian pennywort leaves 100 g
(3$1/2$ oz)

Fenugreek seeds $1/2$ tsp

Cumin seeds $1/2$ tsp

Salt $1/2$ tsp

Bring rice and water to the boil until porridge turns thick and mushy.

Blend (process) coconut milk with Indian pennywort leaves in a blender (processor) until smooth.

Add blended mixture together with remaining ingredients to porridge. Return to the boil and remove from heat. Serve hot.

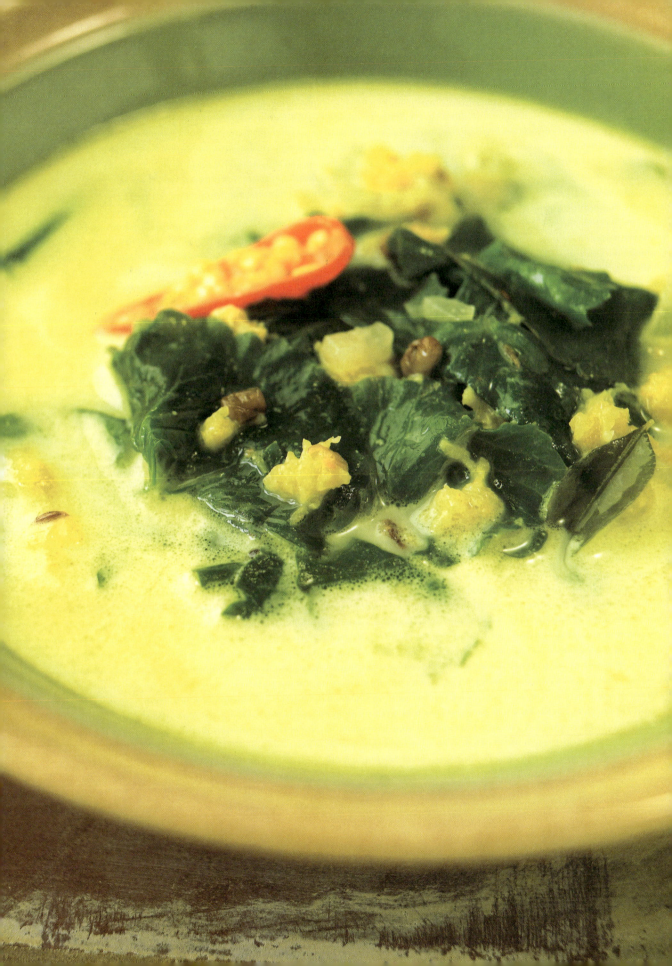

Jackfruit

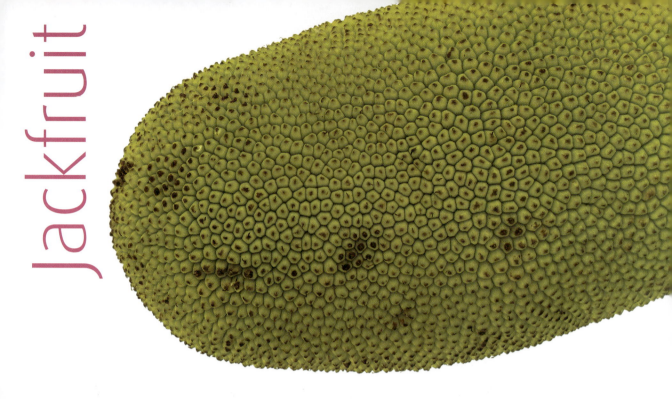

Common Jackfruit
Sanskrit Panasa
Tamil Pala pazham, Pala maram
Botanical Artocarpus heterophyllus

Jackfruit is a large fruit that resembles a pine cone and can weigh up to 10 kg. The interior of the fruit comprises large edible bulbs of yellow flesh containing smooth, oval and brown-coloured seeds. The flesh is sweet with a crunchy texture.

For cooking, the unripe fruit is often used. Before cutting an unripe fruit, coat the knife and your hands with salad oil first to ensure the easy removal of the milky sap from the knife and hands. The bulbs of fruit, with their skins and seeds intact, are boiled in lightly salted water until tender; the cooked bulbs of fruit are then skinned, seeded and served as a vegetable while the edible seeds achieve a tasty, floury texture when cooked.

In traditional healing practices, jackfruit flesh and seeds are a cooling and nutritious food. The seeds are believed to relieve nausea while the dried sap of the fruit when mixed with vinegar is believed to promote the healing of wounds and snake bites. A remedy of the juice of the tender fruit with coconut milk and jaggery is prescribed as an antidote for drug poisoning. Jackfruit leaves, with its antibacterial and calming properties, are used in remedies to treat skin diseases and insomnia.

Insomnia Treatment

Tender jackfruit leaves 10 pieces,
washed and finely shredded

Grated coconut 4 Tbsp

Salt $^1/_4$ tsp

Ground black pepper $^1/_2$ tsp

Combine all ingredients and consume this portion
every evening as required.

Jackfruit Payasam

Preparation time: 15 minutes
Cooking time: 20 minutes
Serves: 5

**Skinned split green (mung) beans
(*moong* dhal)** 250 g (9 oz)

Water 2.5 litres (80 fl oz / 10 cups)

Jaggery 170 g (6 oz)

Thick coconut milk 250 ml
(8 fl oz / 1 cup) (see page 50)

Jackfruit 400 g (14 oz), seeded
and sliced

Cardamom powder 1 tsp

Salt a pinch

Ginger powder $^1/_2$ tsp

Wash beans, drain and put in a deep pot. Add water and
bring to the boil over medium heat until beans are soft
and broken. Reduce heat and simmer.

Boil jaggery in 250 ml (8 fl oz / 1 cup) water until
dissolved. Strain mixture into simmering pot of beans.

Stir in coconut milk, jackfruit slices, cardamom powder,
salt and ginger powder. Return to the boil for 2 minutes.

Remove from heat and serve hot as a dessert. If serving
cold, cool completely before refrigerating for at least
an hour.

FROM LEFT TO RIGHT: *Insomnia Treatment (page 123), Jackfruit Payasam (page 123)*

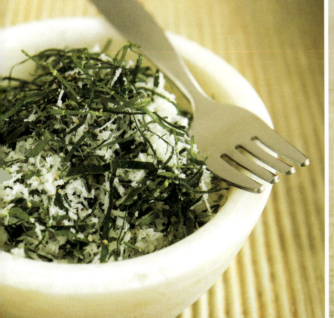
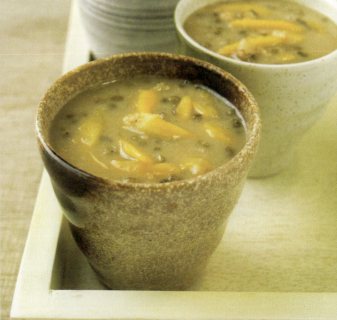

Jaggery

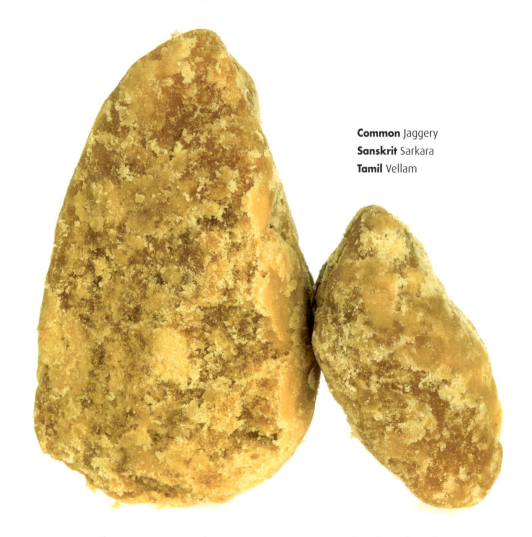

Common Jaggery
Sanskrit Sarkara
Tamil Vellam

Jaggery is a natural sweetener made by boiling sugar cane juice until it becomes a thick paste before it is left to cool and solidify. It tastes similar to dark brown sugar and is sold in the form of large lumps or solid cakes. The colour of jaggery ranges from mustard yellow to reddish-brown, depending on the quality of the sugar canes used. It is sticky and has a crumbly texture.

In Indian cuisine, jaggery is used in the making of chutneys, sweet lentil dishes and some sweets and desserts. In rural India, tea is often sweetened with jaggery instead of sugar. The resulting thick and sweet brew helps to regulate the blood sugar level and also serves as an instant energy-booster for farmers and workmen who require lots of energy in their heavy manual work.

A good source of vitamins A and B, jaggery also contains minerals such as calcium, potassium, sulphur, iron and phosphorus. The natural sweetener has been used by Indians for centuries in Ayurvedic healing. Medicinal treatments include remedies for purifying the blood and relieving rheumatism as well as nausea. It is a healing food that helps regulate the heart and liver functions while stimulating the body's metabolism at the same time. In many Indian homes, jaggery is regarded as the 'medicine sugar' as it is used in simple remedies for common ailments including coughs, indigestion and constipation.

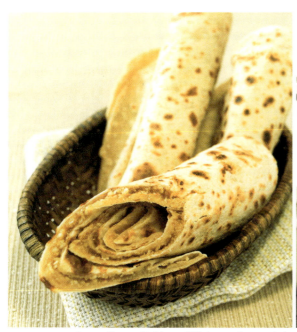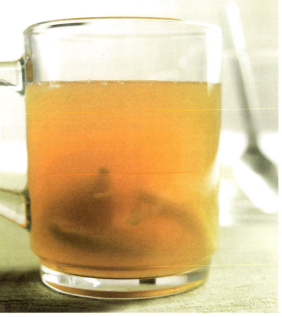

FROM LEFT TO RIGHT: Jaggery Sesame Roti (page 125), Jaggery Lemonade (page 126)

Jaggery Sesame Roti

Preparation time: 20 minutes
Cooking time: 15 minutes
Serves: 6

White sesame seeds 80 g (3 oz)

Jaggery 60 g (2 oz), grated

Salt 1^1/$_4$ tsp

Fine wholewheat flour (*atta* flour) 250 g (9 oz)

Plain (all-purpose) flour 250 g (9 oz)

Ghee (clarified butter) 1 Tbsp

Lukewarm water 350 ml (11^2/$_3$ fl oz/ 1^3/$_8$ cups)

Dry-roast sesame seeds lightly and grind into a coarse mixture.

Put sesame seeds, grated jaggery and ^{1}/$_4$ tsp salt into a mixing bowl and mix well. Set aside.

In a separate mixing bowl, sift both types of flour together with remaining salt.

Add ghee and water to flour mixture, then mix well and knead to form a soft, pliable dough. Divide into 12 equal-sized balls. Roll out each ball into a disc about 14 cm (5.5-in) in diameter.

Spread 1–2 Tbsp sesame and jaggery mixture on 6 of the discs, leaving a 1-cm (^{1}/$_2$-in) border around each disc. Place another disc of dough over these discs and press around the edges to seal.

Fry roti on a non-stick pan on both sides until golden brown. Serve hot as a snack.

Cough and Cold Remedy for Children

Holy basil leaves 20

Crumbled jaggery 1 tsp

Wash leaves thoroughly. Pound to a coarse pulp, then wrap in a piece of clean muslin cloth and squeeze to extract juice.

Mix juice with crumbled jaggery. Let the sick child take this portion thrice a day.

Jaggery Lemonade

Preparation time: 10 minutes
Cooking time: 5 minutes
Serves: 4

Jaggery 160 g (5^1/$_2$ oz), grated

Ginger 3-cm (1^1/$_2$-in) knob, peeled and pounded

Salt ^{1}/$_4$ tsp

Water 500 ml (16 fl oz / 2 cups)

White peppercorns 1 tsp, coarsely pounded

Freshly squeezed lemon juice 200 ml (6^2/$_3$ fl oz / ^{3}/$_4$ cup)

Lemon 2 or 3 slices (optional)

Put all ingredients, except lemon juice and lemon slices into a pot. Bring to the boil for 5 minutes.

Stir in lemon juice and add lemon slices, if using. Serve hot as a soothing drink.

If serving chilled, strain mixture and stir in lemon juice, then cool completely and add lemon slices, if using. Refrigerate until ready to serve.

Relief for Menstrual Cramps

Bitter gourd leaves 50 g (2 oz)

Black peppercorns 3

Garlic 1 clove, peeled

Grated jaggery 1 tsp

Grind all ingredients together into a paste and take this portion once a day during menstruation to relieve menstrual cramps.

Remedy for Swollen Feet during Pregnancy

Fennel seeds 2 tsp, lightly pounded

Grated jaggery 1 tsp

Water 250 ml (8 fl oz / 1 cup)

Bring all ingredients to the boil until liquid is reduced to about 125 ml (4 fl oz / ^{1}/$_2$ cup).

Strain liquid and drink this portion at least thrice a day or until swelling of the feet subsides.

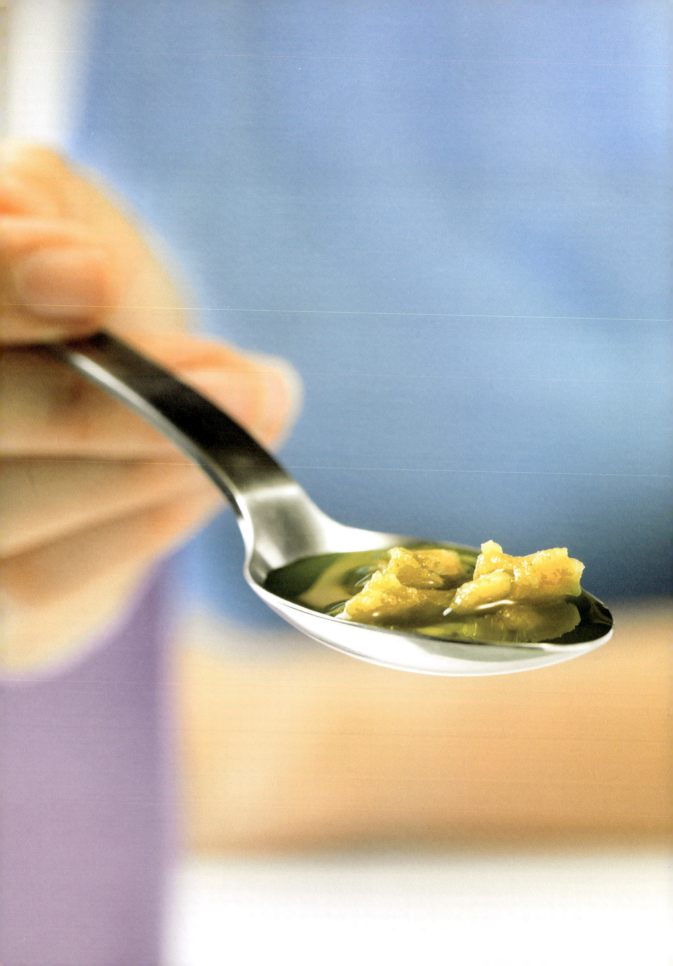

Lemon and Lime

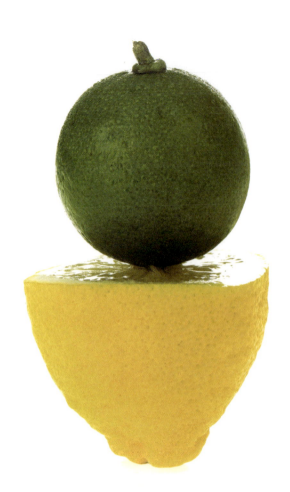

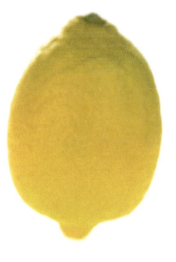

Common Lemon
Sanskrit Ruchaka, Nimbaka, Vijapura
Tamil Elumichai, Sidalai
Botanical Citrus limon

Common Lime
Sanskrit Surabhi nimbu
Tamil Elumichankaai, Narthai
Botanical Citrus aurantifolia

Lemons and limes are very similar in flavour and healing properties; they are regarded as good substitutes for each other in Indian cuisine and healing practices. With their strong antibacterial and antioxidant properties, the citrus fruits are also common ingredients in home beauty treatments. In the kitchen, lemons and limes add a tangy flavour to many Indian dishes including curries, pickles and salads.

In terms of medicinal treatments, a daily drink of vitamin-C rich lemon or lime juice with warm water is useful for regulating one's bowel movement and also serves as a good preventative measure against the common cold. The fruit juices are often used to make cooling drinks for bringing down fevers or quenching thirst. Pickled lemons or limes are popular home remedies for stimulating sluggish appetites as well as relieving stomach disorders such as indigestion and bloating. The essential oil, limonene, which resides in the fruit peels is popularly used in natural remedies to treat muscle cramps, gout and arthritis as the oil stimulates the flow of lymphatic fluids in the body.

Lemon Apple Remedy for Diarrhoea

Red apple 1, peeled and cored
Lemon juice 2 Tbsp
Honey 1 Tbsp
Cinnamon powder $^1/_2$ tsp

Blend (process) apple to a coarse mixture in the blender (processor).

Mix in remaining ingredients. Consume this portion immediately to stop diarrhoea.

Lime Pickle

Preparation time: 15 minutes
Cooking time: 10 minutes
Makes: 1 x 750 ml jar

Ripe limes 500 g (1 lb 1$^1/_2$ oz)
Salt 40 g (1$^1/_2$ oz)
Gingelly oil 300 ml (10 fl oz / 1$^1/_4$ cups)
Fenugreek seeds 1 Tbsp
Black mustard seeds 3$^1/_2$ tsp
Chilli powder 80 g (3 oz)
Asafoetida powder 1$^1/_2$ tsp
Curry leaves 3 sprigs, stems discarded and shredded
Young ginger 150 g (5$^1/_3$ oz), peeled and minced

Cut each lime into 8 wedges. Rub lime wedges with salt and store in a large, airtight glass jar for 3 days, tossing often.

Heat 1 Tbsp oil and fry fenugreek and 2 tsp mustard seeds until aromatic. Cool thoroughly, then pound coarsely with mortar and pestle.

Stir pounded spice mixture, chilli and asafoetida powders into jar of salted limes and combine well.

Heat remaining oil and fry remaining mustard seeds until aromatic. Add curry leaves and ginger and sauté for 1 minute. Transfer to jar of lime pickle. Mix well and cool thoroughly before closing the jar.

Refrigerate for at least 10 days before serving with rice and other dishes. If refrigerated, pickle keeps well for up to a year.

FROM LEFT TO RIGHT: *Lemon Apple Remedy for Diarrhoea (page 129), Lime Pickle (page 129)*

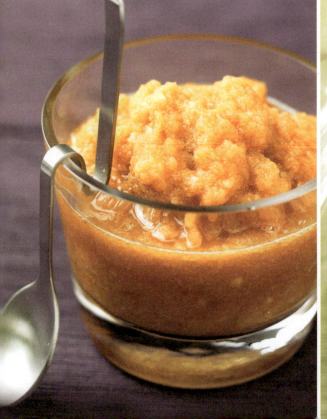
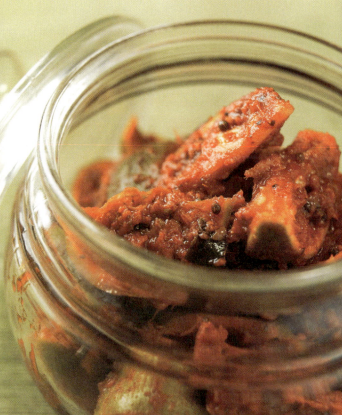

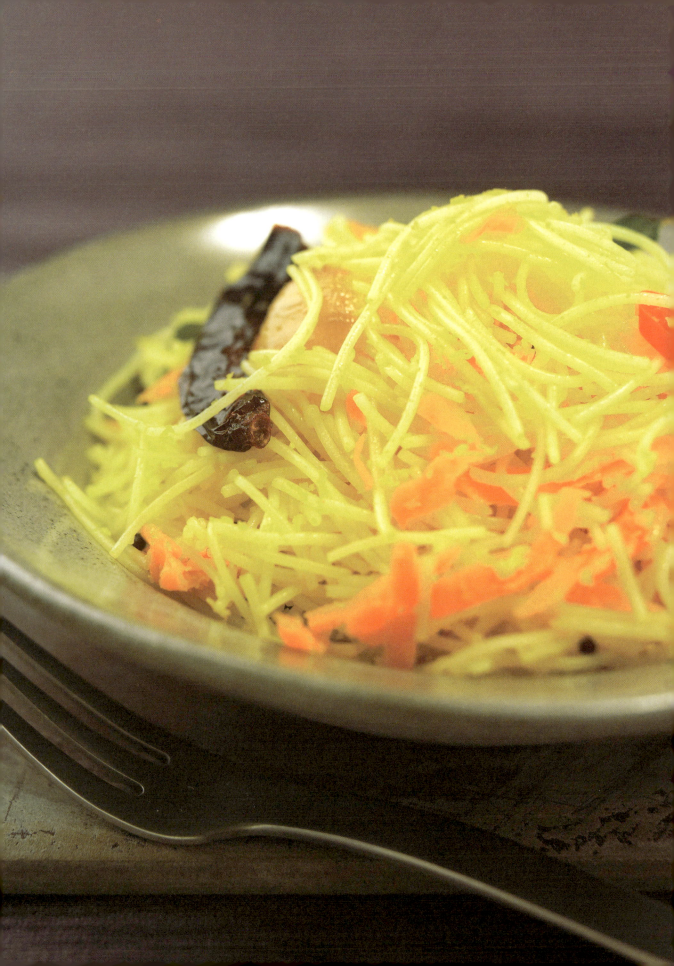

Home-made Brass Polish

Lime or lemon juice 3 Tbsp

Salt 1 Tbsp

Mix all ingredients together and use it to scrub dull brass ornaments or utensils. See how they shine after a good scrub and polish!

Wrinkle Eraser

Apply this oil often and see your wrinkles disappear. This same mixture is also excellent for treating scalp conditions such as dandruff. Dancers can keep their joints pliant by massaging their joints with this oil too.

Lemon juice 1 Tbsp

Almond or gingelly oil 1 Tbsp

Place all ingredients into a small bowl. Using a fork, whisk until an emulsion is formed.

Gently massage oil onto the part of skin with wrinkles or deep lines. Leave on for 20 minutes, then rinse off with warm water and pat dry with a clean towel.

Remedy for Cough

Ginger 3-cm (1^1/$_2$-in) knob, peeled and grated

Lemon or lime ^{1}/$_2$, thinly sliced

Garlic 1 clove, peeled and crushed

Water 500 ml (16 fl oz / 2 cups)

Honey to taste

Place all ingredients except honey into a pot. Bring to the boil, then reduce heat and simmer for 15 minutes.

Strain, stir in honey to taste and serve hot.

Lemon Vermicelli

Preparation time: 15 minutes
Cooking time: 10 minutes
Serves: 6

Dried rice vermicelli 600 g (1 lb 5 oz)

Cooking oil 3 Tbsp

Black mustard seeds 1^1/$_2$ tsp

Dried chillies 3, cut into 2-cm (1-in) pieces

Onions 2, medium, peeled and finely sliced

Red chillies 3, sliced

Curry leaves 2 sprigs, stems discarded

Carrot 200 g (7 oz), peeled and coarsely grated

Turmeric powder ^{1}/$_2$ tsp

Salt 2 tsp

Lemon juice 50 ml (1^2/$_3$ fl oz / ^{1}/$_4$ cup)

Grated coconut 100 g (3^1/$_2$ oz), steamed for 10 minutes

Soak vermicelli in water for 20 minutes. Drain and pour in boiling water, then soak until dried vermicelli is soft and cooked. Drain in a colander and refresh with running water until vermicelli is no longer warm. Set aside.

Heat oil and fry mustard seeds and dried chillies until mustard seeds stop spluttering.

Add onions, chillies and curry leaves and sauté until onions turn golden brown.

Add grated carrot and turmeric powder and sauté for 1 minute.

Add remaining ingredients including vermicelli and stir-fry over high heat until well combined. Serve hot as a light meal on its own or with other dishes.

Lotus Root

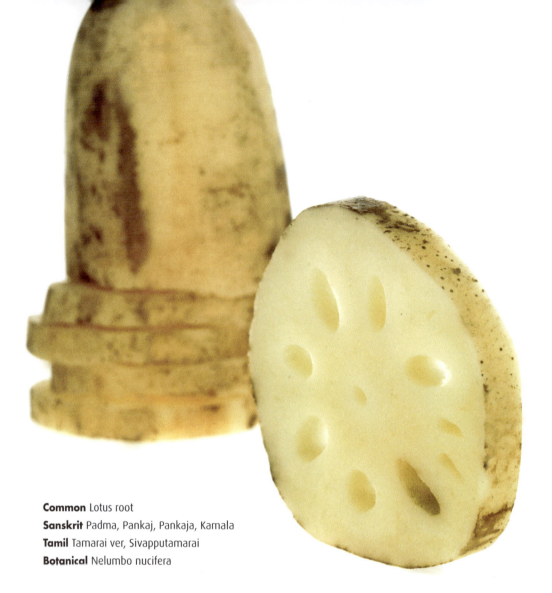

Common Lotus root
Sanskrit Padma, Pankaj, Pankaja, Kamala
Tamil Tamarai ver, Sivapputamarai
Botanical Nelumbo nucifera

Smooth-skinned and large, lotus roots are the swollen stems of the lotus plant; they grow in sections and are shaped like sausage links. The crisp flesh of the root has a mildly pleasant flavour and is as densely-textured as new potatoes. In Indian cuisine, lotus roots are cooked in a wide variety of dishes including stews, pickles and soups; lotus roots are even used by some as a substitute for meat.

To prepare lotus roots for cooking, separate the sections and wash thoroughly. Slice off and discard the 'necks' between each section before peeling off the skins. As the stems discolour quickly, soak the pieces of lotus root in cold water until ready for use.

In traditional healing practices, raw lotus root juice is believed to be cooling for the system and to help in promoting good blood circulation. To stop wounds or cuts from bleeding, applying a poultice of crushed raw lotus root is believed to be effective. Eating cooked lotus roots can help stimulate the production of red blood cells in the body; they are especially beneficial for anaemic women who suffer from heavy menstruation as well as for persons who have lost large amounts of blood due to serious injuries. Other traditional medicinal purposes include treatments for phlegmy coughs and colds, diarrhoea, stomach ulcers, gastritis and haemorrhoids.

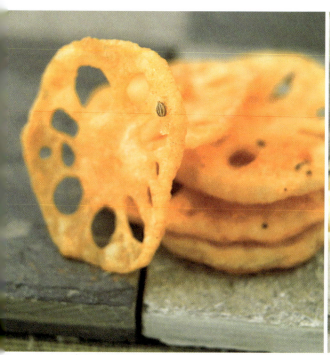 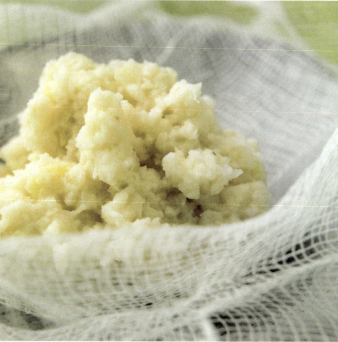

FROM LEFT TO RIGHT: Lotus Root Fritters (page 133), Lotus Root Plaster for Nasal Congestion (page 135)

Lotus Root Fritters

Preparation time: 10 minutes
Cooking time: 15 minutes
Serves: 5

Lotus root 500 g (1lb 1¹/₂ oz), washed and scrubbed clean

Rice flour 300 g (10¹/₂ oz)

Water 300 ml (10 fl oz / 1¹/₄ cups)

Ajwain seeds 1 tsp

Chilli powder 1 tsp

Salt 1 tsp

Black peppercorns 1 tsp, coarsely pounded

Cooking oil for deep-frying

Slice lotus root very thinly crossways and soak in water to prevent slices from turning brown. Set aside.

Combine rice flour, water, ajwain seeds, chilli powder, salt and black peppercorns together to form a batter.

Drain lotus root slices and pat dry with absorbent paper towels. Dip in prepared batter and deep-fry in hot oil until golden brown.

Drain on absorbent paper towels and serve hot as a snack.

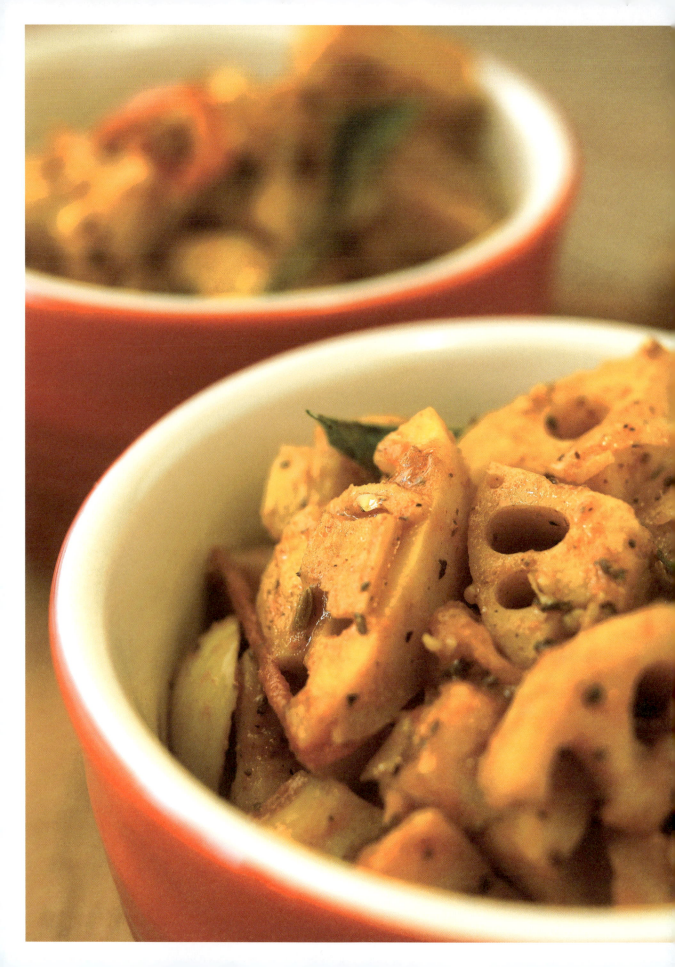

Lotus Root Plaster for Nasal Congestion

This mixture helps to draw mucus from the nose and throat if one suffers from nasal congestion.

Freshly grated lotus root 100 g (3^1/$_2$ oz)
Freshly grated ginger 1 Tbsp
Plain (all-purpose) flour 2 Tbsp
Water 1 Tbsp

Mix all ingredients together in a stainless steel or porcelain bowl.

Spread a thick layer of paste on a piece of clean gauze, then place directly on the throat or nose, paste side facing down, for about 20 minutes, until mixture dries up a little. Repeat a few times daily until mucus subsides.

Black Pepper Lotus Root

Preparation time: 20 minutes
Cooking time: 15 minutes
Serves: 8

Lotus root 750 g (1 lb 10 oz), washed and scrubbed
Water for boiling
Turmeric powder 1 tsp
Coconut oil 2 Tbsp
Fennel seeds 1^1/$_2$ tsp
Cumin seeds 1 tsp
Black peppercorns 2 Tbsp, coarsely pounded
Onions 4, large, peeled and thinly sliced
Ginger 2-cm (1-in) knob, peeled and julienned
Garlic 7 cloves, peeled and thinly sliced
Curry leaves 2 sprigs, stems discarded
Tomatoes 2, medium, chopped
Meat curry powder 1 Tbsp
Salt 1^1/$_2$ tsp
Water 250 ml (8 fl oz / 1 cup)

Cut lotus root into 1-cm (^{1}/$_2$-in) thick slices crossways, then cut each slice into quarters.

Bring water to the boil, then add lotus root and turmeric powder and boil until lotus root is tender, about 5 minutes. Drain in a colander and set aside.

Heat oil and fry fennel and cumin seeds until aromatic. Add black peppercorns and sauté for 1 minute. Add onions and ginger and sauté until onions turn golden brown.

Add garlic, curry leaves and tomatoes and fry until tomatoes turn pulpy.

Add curry powder, salt and water. Cook over low heat until oil separates.

Add lotus root pieces and cook, stirring occasionally until gravy is almost dry. Serve hot with rice.

Lotus Root Tea

This tea helps to decongest and eliminate mucus from the nasal passages and lungs if one has a phlegmy cough and cold.

Lotus root 1 section, about 5-cm (2^1/$_2$-in) long, washed, scrubbed and grated
Freshly squeezed ginger juice 1 Tbsp
Water
Black salt a pinch

Wrap grated lotus root in a piece of clean muslin cloth and squeeze to extract juice.

Pour lotus root juice into a measuring cup and add ginger juice. Add water equal to amount of liquid in measuring cup.

Transfer liquid to a pot and bring to the boil. Stir in salt, remove from heat and drink.

Mango

A popular fruit, the mango is known for its saccharine sweet, juicy flesh when ripe. When handling mangoes, be careful to wipe off any residual milky sap on the fruit, as it may cause an itch. In India, mangoes have a mind-boggling variety of culinary uses. Ripe mangoes are made into spiced pickles and drinks; partially ripe or green mangoes are peeled and used as fillings for pies or cooked in curries and jellies. Green mangoes are also popularly used in making chutneys. In North India, unripe mangoes are dried and ground into a sour-tasting powder known as *amchur*.

Common Mango
Sanskrit Aamra, Amra
Tamil Mangai (raw), Mampazham (ripe)
Botanical Mangifera indica

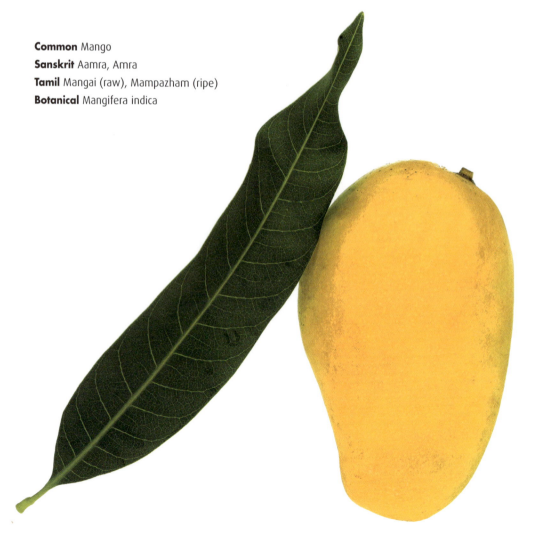

Apart from its culinary uses, the mango is perceived to have great medicinal value in India. Consuming the fruit helps treat beriberi. A mixture of mango pulp and honey is a favourite home remedy for bronchitis. For treating scabies, rub the pulp on affected skin to aid the healing process. The fruit is also a diuretic which helps eliminate toxins in the body through the urine. Fibre-rich mangoes are similarly effective in the treatment of constipation and haemorrhoids.

For night blindness caused by a deficiency in vitamin A, a diet of ripe mangoes rich in vitamin A is highly beneficial.

Consuming mangoes on a regular basis is also believed to keep the skin soft and supple as mangoes are rich in antioxidants. However, unripe mangoes, with their high acid content, must not be consumed in excess as this may cause throat irritation and indigestion.

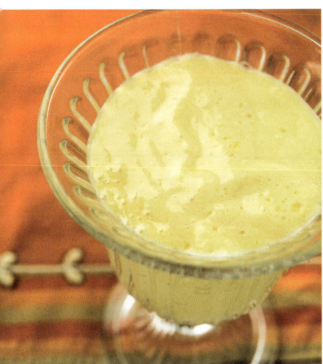 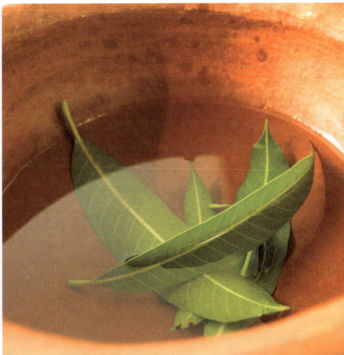

FROM LEFT TO RIGHT: *Mango Lassi (page 137), Remedy for the Treatment of Early Diabetes (page 138)*

Mango Lassi

Preparation time: 10 minutes
Serves: 2

Natural yoghurt 300 ml
 (10 fl oz / 1 1/4 cups)

Lemon juice 1/2 tsp

Ripe mangoes 2, peeled, seeded and
 cut into pieces

Cold water or milk 85 ml
 (2 1/2 fl oz / 1/3 cup)

Honey 4 Tbsp

Ice cubes 9–10, standard-sized

Blend all ingredients except ice cubes in a blender (processor) until honey has dissolved and mixture, smooth.

Add ice cubes and blend until frothy. Serve this drink immediately.

Remedy for the Treatment of Early Diabetes

Believed to lower blood sugar levels, the tender leaves of the mango tree are considered useful in controlling early diabetes.

Tender mango leaves 10

Water 400 ml (13^{1}/$_{3}$ fl oz / 1^{5}/$_{8}$ cups)

Wash mango leaves well to remove any traces of pesticide. Soak leaves in water overnight.

Squeeze leaves well to extract all moisture, then strain liquid and drink this portion daily to control early diabetes.

Remedy for Reducing Blood Sugar Levels

Tender mango leaves 50

Water

Wash leaves well and wipe dry thoroughly.

Place them on a clean sheet of muslin cloth and dry in the shade.

When completely dry, grind into a powder and store in an airtight container.

Mix ^{1}/$_{2}$ tsp powder with 250 ml (8 fl oz /1 cup) water and consume this portion twice daily to help lower one's blood sugar level.

Chettinad Fish Curry

Preparation time: 20 minutes
Cooking time: 20 minutes
Serves: 7

Cooking oil 3 Tbsp

Skinned split black lentils (*urad* dhal) ^{1}/$_{2}$ tsp

Black peppercorns ^{1}/$_{2}$ tsp

Fenugreek seeds 1^{1}/$_{2}$ tsp

Black mustard seeds 1 tsp

Shallots 100 g (3^{1}/$_{2}$ oz), peeled and sliced

Garlic 10 cloves, peeled and sliced

Curry leaves 2 sprigs, stems discarded

Tomatoes 3, sliced

Tamarind pulp 250 g (9 oz), mixed with 1.75 litres (56 fl oz / 7 cups) water and strained

Salt 1^{1}/$_{2}$ tsp

Unripe mangoes 3, skins left on, seeded and cut into 1.5-cm (^{3}/$_{4}$-in) slices

Fish fillet 1 kg (2 lbs 3 oz), sliced

Chopped coriander (cilantro) leaves 3 Tbsp

Spice Paste

Chilli powder 4 Tbsp

Coriander (cilantro) powder 4 Tbsp

Cumin powder 1 Tbsp

Turmeric powder 1 tsp

Ground fennel seeds 2 tsp

Water 400 ml (13^{1}/$_{3}$ fl oz/ 1^{5}/$_{8}$ cups)

Put ingredients for spice paste into large bowl and combine well.

Heat oil and fry lentils until golden brown. Add peppercorns, fenugreek and mustard seeds and fry until aromatic.

Add shallots, garlic and curry leaves and sauté until shallots turn golden brown. Add tomatoes and sauté until they turn pulpy.

Add prepared spice paste and fry over low heat until oil separates. Pour in tamarind juice and add mango slices.

Simmer over medium heat for about 10 minutes, or until oil separates.

Add fish slices and coriander leaves, then simmer until fish is cooked. Serve with rice or bread.

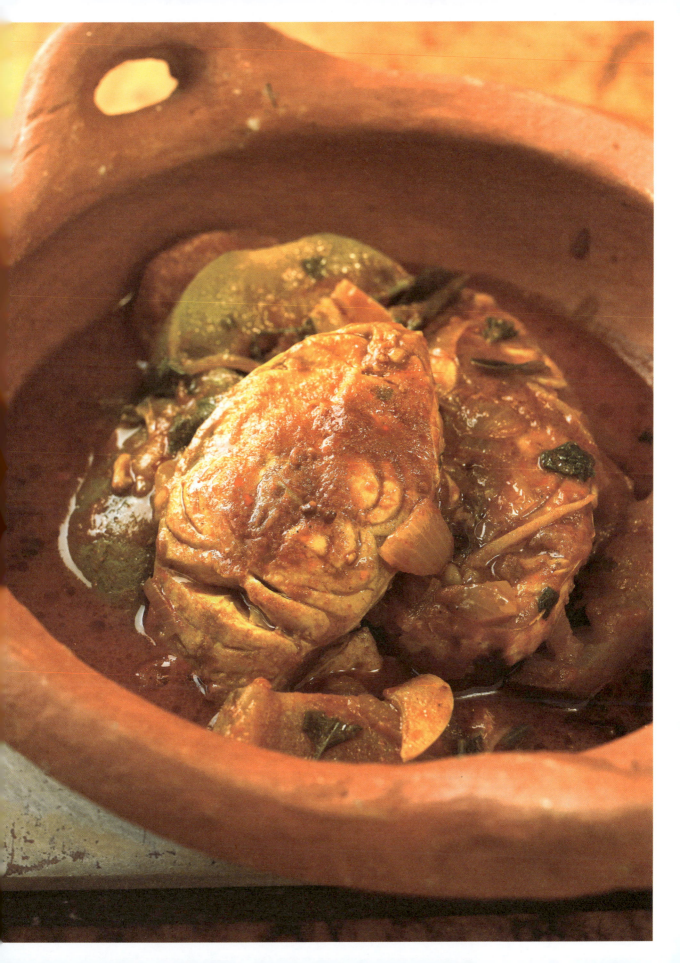

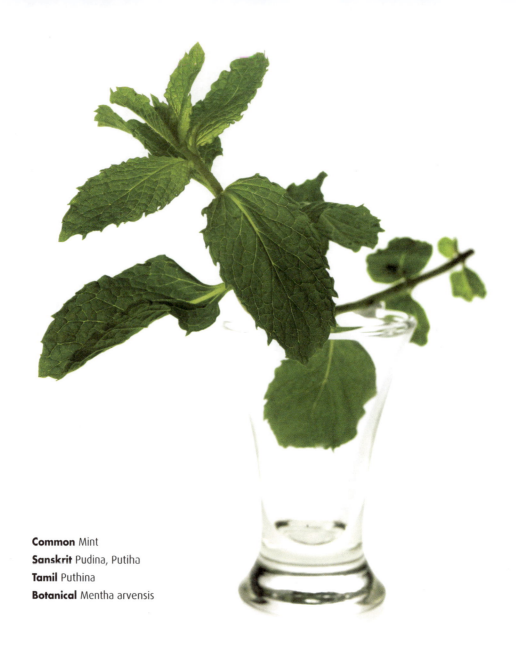

Mint

Common Mint
Sanskrit Pudina, Putiha
Tamil Puthina
Botanical Mentha arvensis

A herb that has pointed, bright green leaves with jagged edges. The fresh fragrant leaves impart a mildly sweet and cool taste to the mouth because of the menthol content in the plant.

Mint is cultivated in India for use in many culinary preparations as well as healing practices. The oil extracted from the plant is highly regarded for its antibacterial, anaesthetic and pain-relieving properties. It is used in the manufacture of many medicinal products including ointments, creams and cough syrups. In traditional Indian healing, mint has been used in remedies to treat many ailments including headaches, colds, flu, colic and flatulence.

Mint is also a useful herb for alleviating morning sickness in pregnant women. It is even gentle enough for use in remedies for colicky babies. For external treatments, the oil is rubbed onto affected parts to treat muscle cramps and aches. A fresh infusion of mint leaves helps soothe the stomach as well as relieve flatulence and a bloated feeling.

Pudina Rice

Preparation time: 15 minutes
Cooking time: 15 minutes
Serves: 6

Cooking oil 1¹/₂ Tbsp

Cinnamon stick 1, 3-cm (1¹/₂-in) long

Cardamoms 5

Cloves 5

Onion 1, medium, peeled and sliced

Mint leaves 80 g (3 oz), chopped

Coriander (cilantro) leaves 50 g (2 oz), chopped

Tomatoes 2, chopped

Basmati rice 600 g (1 lb 5 oz), washed and drained

Salt 1¹/₂ tsp

Cumin powder 1 tsp

Turmeric powder ¹/₂ tsp

Thick coconut milk 1 litre (32 fl oz / 4 cups) (see page 50)

Spice Blend

Onion 1, medium, coarsely chopped

Garlic cloves 8 cloves, peeled and left whole

Ginger 3-cm (1¹/₂-in) knob, peeled

Green chillies 2

Blend (process) ingredients for spice blend in a blender (processor) until smooth.

Heat oil and fry cinnamon, cardamoms and cloves until aromatic. Add onion and sauté until golden brown.

Add chopped mint and coriander leaves and tomatoes, then sauté until tomatoes turn soft. Transfer to the electric rice cooker.

Add prepared spice blend, rice, salt, cumin and turmeric powders and coconut milk. Stir to combine well.

Switch on rice cooker and cook rice. When ready, serve with salad or pickle and other dishes.

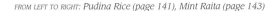

FROM LEFT TO RIGHT: *Pudina Rice (page 141), Mint Raita (page 143)*

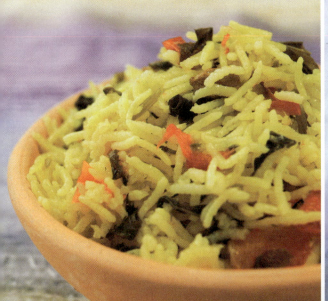
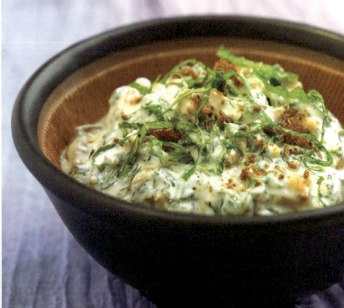

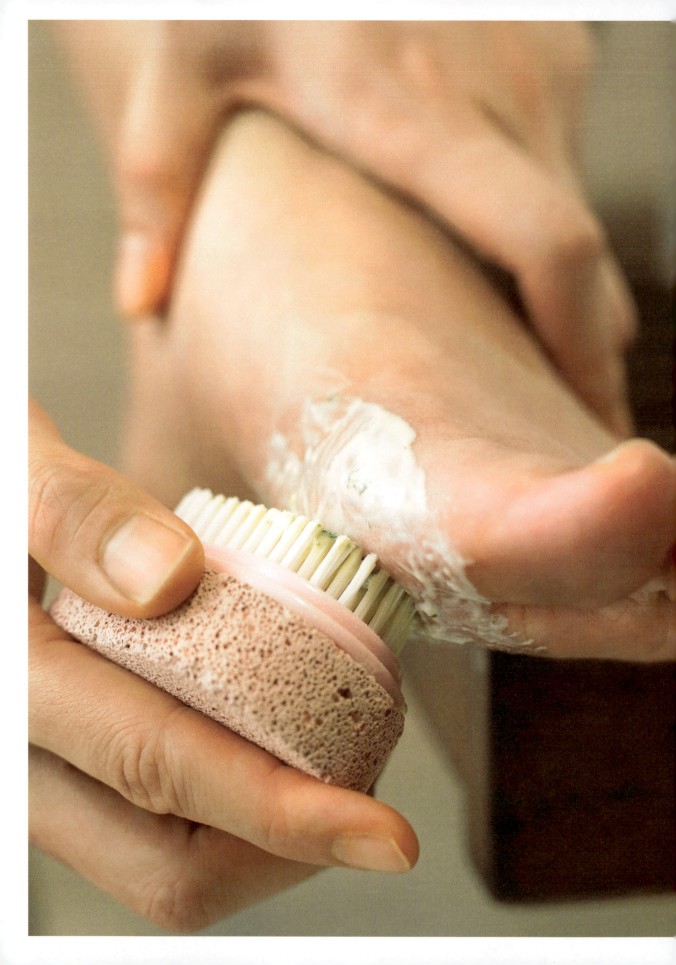

Mint Raita

Preparation time: 10 minutes
Cooking time: 5
Serves: 6

Cumin seeds 1¹/₂ tsp

Natural yoghurt 400 ml
(13¹/₃ fl oz/ 1⁵/₈ cups)

Salt 1 tsp

Raisins 60 g (2 oz), chopped

Mint leaves 80 g (3 oz), very
finely chopped

Dry-roast cumin seeds until aromatic and
pound coarsely.

Put yoghurt, salt and cumin seeds into a mixing bowl
and whisk with a fork until smooth.

Add remaining ingredients and combine well.
Serve chilled with rice or bread and other dishes.

Mint Tea

Drink this tea to get rid of nausea. The menthol in mint soothes the lining of the digestive tract
and stimulates the production of bile, which is an essential digestive fluid. A hot cup of herbal tea
is an excellent way to settle your stomach after a big meal.

Fresh mint leaves 10

Boiling water 250 ml (8 fl oz / 1 cup)

Honey to taste

Wash leaves and place into cup. Pour boiling water over
and steep for 10 minutes.

Strain liquid and stir in honey to taste. Serve hot.

*Note: Add a pinch of ground anise, caraway or cinnamon to increase the
effectiveness of the tea as a breath freshener.*

Relaxing Foot Scrub

After a tiring day, there is nothing like a minty food scrub. Indulge in this highly soothing and
relaxing treatment.

Natural yoghurt 250 ml (8 fl oz / 1 cup)

Coarse salt 125 g (4¹/₂ oz)

Mint leaves 100 g (3¹/₂ oz), pounded

Mix all ingredients together.

Apply onto feet and very gently scrub all the rough spots.
Rinse and pat dry with a clean towel. Follow with the
application of moisturiser.

Neem

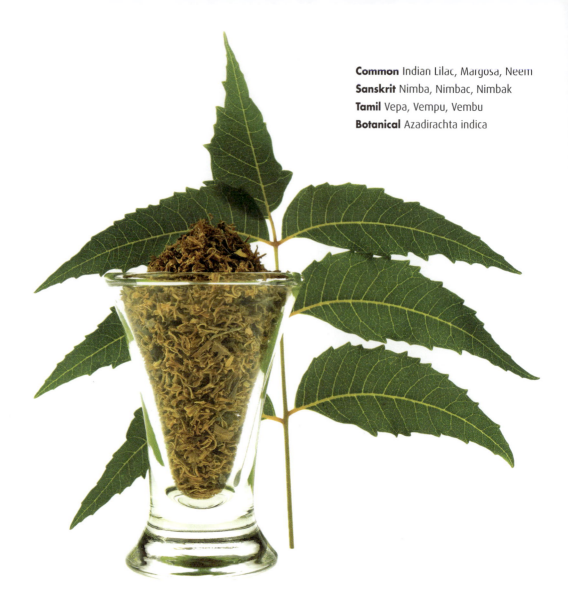

Common Indian Lilac, Margosa, Neem
Sanskrit Nimba, Nimbac, Nimbak
Tamil Vepa, Vempu, Vembu
Botanical Azadirachta indica

Native to Northeast India, the neem tree has pointed, sharply serrated leaves which are extremely bitter in taste and fragrant white flowers. Neem is highly valued in India for its multitude of healing properties.

In South Indian cuisine, the flowers of the neem tree are used for cooking a thin, spicy soup known as *rasam*. It is said that taking this soup once a week is beneficial to one's general physical well-being and helps ward off the onset of any diseases. In some parts of India, neem leaves are served in dishes during celebrations of the New Year to symbolise both the sweet and bitter experiences of the upcoming year.

Medicinally, neem leaves are known to bring down fevers and fight the infection of diseases and speed up the process of recovery. Neem is reported to be effective in the treatment of skin diseases such as ringworm and athlete's foot which affect the scalp and body, intestinal tract disorders and fungal infections of the lungs.

For centuries in rural India, villagers have been chewing on neem twigs to maintain their oral hygiene. The astringent and antiseptic qualities of the tree bark helped keep tooth decay at bay, removed bad breath and prevented the bleeding of gums in the days before toothbrushes and toothpastes became readily available. Neem leaves are also dried and ground into a powder; it is used for cleaning teeth and massaging aching gums. For clear and supple skin, simply massage the body with neem oil or bathe with water in which a handful of freshly crushed neem leaves have been added. For external use, neem leaves are ground into a paste and applied topically on the affected areas such as warts. It is also a common practice among many Indians to gather neem leaves and place them on the beds of those suffering from chicken pox as it is believed that lying on the leaves will help stop the itch that often accompanies chicken pox and also allows the patients to heal faster.

In India, people scatter fresh neem leaves near the beds of those suffering from flu or fever; it is believed that the leaves help to disinfect the air in the room naturally and therefore prevent the spread of the illness. The neem tree is of such great importance in India that the various parts of the tree are used for almost all occasions, from everyday living to sacred occasions. In many villages, neem wood is used as a cooking fuel and also as timber for the construction of roofs. Grains and lentils are stored in containers with neem leaves to keep out insects. During wedding ceremonies at Hindu temples, neem leaves are scattered on the floor to cleanse the air. For funerals, neem branches are used to cover the corpses before they are cremated in pyres.

Remedy for Minor Sprains and Bruises

Fresh neem leaves 150 g (5¹/₃ oz)

Grind neem leaves into a paste with a little water. Apply paste onto affected area and wrap around with a piece of clean muslin cloth or cotton gauze.

Change wrap every 2 hours until sprain or bruise subsides.

Neem Flower Tuvayal

Preparation time: 5 minutes
Cooking time: 10 minutes
Serves: 5

Cooking oil 1 Tbsp

Skinned split black lentils (urad dhal) 1¹/₂ Tbsp

Dried chillies 4, cut into 1-cm (¹/₂-in) pieces

Dried neem flowers 80 g (3 oz)

Instant tamarind paste 2 tsp

Salt ¹/₂ tsp

Heat oil and fry lentils until golden brown. Add dried chillies and fry until they turn a shade darker. Transfer to a plate.

In the same oil, fry neem flowers and tamarind paste until aromatic. Set aside to cool completely.

Blend (process) all ingredients in a blender (processor) without adding water. Serve with rice and other dishes.

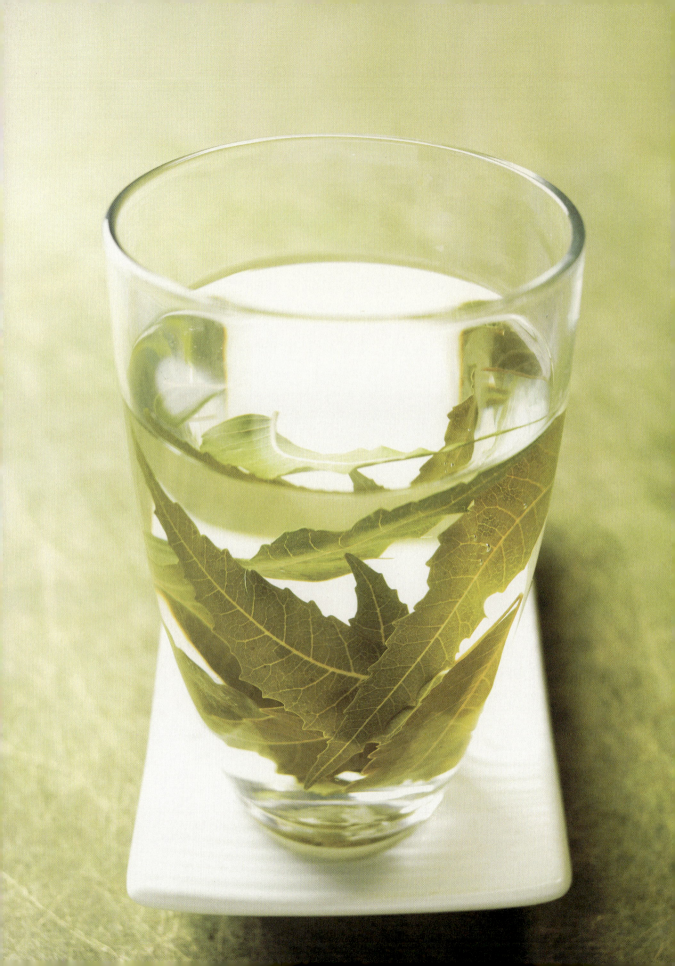

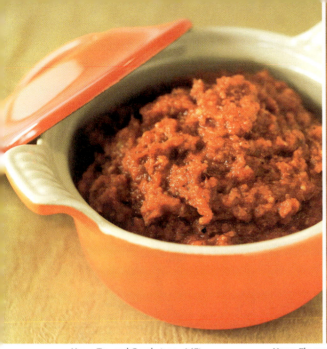
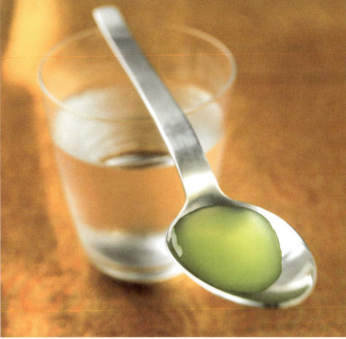

OPPOSITE: Neem Tea and Gargle (page 147) FROM LEFT TO RIGHT: Neem Flower Chutney (page 147), Remedy for Healthy Gums (page 147)

Neem Tea and Gargle

This tea is good for general well-being. Drinking this tea regularly helps in lowering the blood sugar level too. This remedy can also be used as a gargle for achieving healthy gums and fresh breath. Simply cool tea completely and gargle as usual.

Fresh neem leaves 15

Water 250 ml (8 fl oz / 1 cup)

Boil all ingredients together for 1 minute.

Strain liquid and drink this portion twice a day.

Note: To treat a dry cough, serve this tea mixed with 2 tsp honey or add 10 crushed black peppercorns when boiling mixture.

Neem Flower Chutney

Preparation time: 15 minutes
Cooking time: 5 minutes
Serves: 5

Tamarind pulp 100 g (3¹/₂ oz), mixed with 300 ml (10 fl oz / 1¹/₄ cups) water and strained

Grated jaggery 100 g (3¹/₂ oz)

Unripe mango 300 g (10¹/₂ oz), peeled, stoned and cubed

Chilli powder 1 tsp

Salt 1 tsp

Dried neem flowers 3 Tbsp

Bring tamarind juice and jaggery to the boil and simmer until jaggery dissolves. Remove from heat and strain liquid.

Boil strained liquid with mango cubes, chilli powder, salt and neem flowers until mango cubes turn soft. Remove from heat.

Cool thoroughly and serve with rice and other dishes.

Note: This chutney can be stored in sterilised, airtight glass jars for up to a year when refrigerated.

Remedy for Healthy Gums

Freshly squeezed neem juice from pounded leaves 1 Tbsp

Drink 1 Tbsp juice daily for healthy gums.

Onion and Shallot

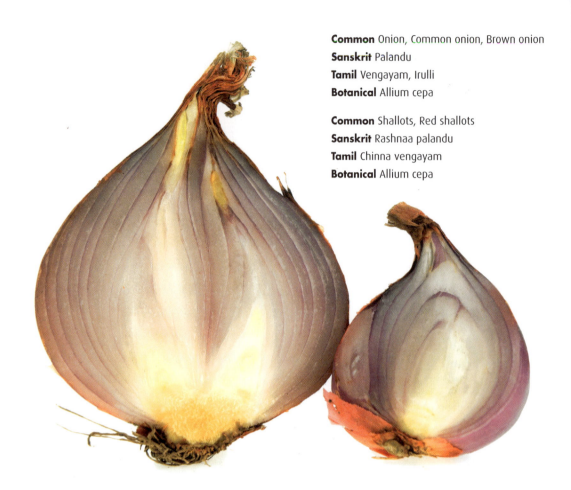

Common Onion, Common onion, Brown onion
Sanskrit Palandu
Tamil Vengayam, Irulli
Botanical Allium cepa

Common Shallots, Red shallots
Sanskrit Rashnaa palandu
Tamil Chinna vengayam
Botanical Allium cepa

Onions and shallots are probably among the earliest cultivated crops in India as they can be stored for a long time or even pickled for future consumption. These underground bulbs of plants which belong to the lily family are widely used in Indian cooking and are popular as spices because of their pungent flavours.

Besides being a rich source of vitamins and minerals such as vitamin C, potassium, calcium and iron, onions and shallots are also high in fibre and do not contain any fat. Medicinally, the bulbs are known to have antibacterial properties and are used in traditional remedies for reducing fevers and healing wounds. The pungent spices are also commonly used in natural treatments for stomach and intestinal disorders as they are believed to remove excessive mucus in the stomach. Used externally, the spices are known for their pain-relieving qualities and are used in remedies for insect bites, minor burns as well as rheumatism. Onions and shallots can also be used to lower blood sugar levels and are effective in treating diabetes.

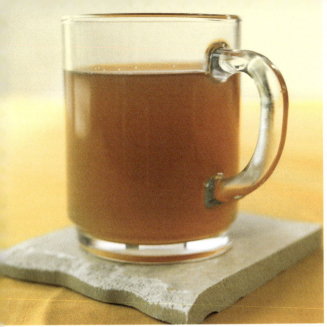
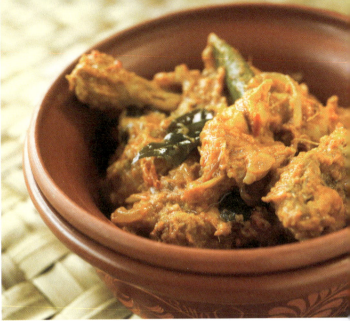

FROM LEFT TO RIGHT: *Shallot Tea (page 149), Onion Chicken (page 149)*

Shallot Tea

This remedy is great for removing flatulence.

Shallots 100 g (3¹/₂ oz), peeled and left whole

Black peppercorns 1 tsp

Garlic 2 cloves, peeled and left whole

Water 1 litre (32 fl oz / 4 cups)

Sugar 1 tsp

Salt ¹/₄ tsp

Using mortar and pestle, pound shallots, peppercorns and garlic coarsely.

Put pounded ingredients into a pot and add water, sugar and salt. Bring to the boil and simmer for 10 minutes.

Remove from heat, strain liquid and serve hot.

Onion Chicken

Preparation time: 1 hour
Cooking time: 20 minutes
Serves: 6

Chicken 1, medium, skinned and cut into 10 pieces

Ghee (clarified butter) 2 Tbsp

Green chillies 2, sliced

Onions 4, peeled and finely chopped

Tomatoes 2, medium, finely chopped

Ginger paste 2 Tbsp

Garlic paste 2 Tbsp

Meat curry powder 2 Tbsp

Chilli powder 1 tsp

Salt 1¹/₂ tsp

Marinade

Natural yoghurt 200 ml (6²/₃ fl oz / ³/₄ cup)

Coriander (cilantro) leaves 100 g (3¹/₂ oz), blended (processed) into a paste

Onions 4, medium, peeled and cut into rings

To marinate chicken, make slits on the surface of chicken pieces, and rub yoghurt and coriander paste all over. Mix in onion rings and set aside for 60 minutes.

In a non-stick pan, cover and cook chicken over low heat, lifting lid to stir occasionally until chicken is almost cooked. Set aside.

In a separate large pan, heat ghee and sauté green chillies and onions until onions turn light brown. Add tomatoes and sauté until soft.

Add ginger and garlic pastes, curry and chilli powders and salt, then fry over low heat until oil separates.

Add chicken pieces and cook, stirring occasionally for about 20 minutes, or until chicken pieces are fully cooked and well-coated with gravy. Serve hot with rice and other dishes.

Pepper

Common Pepper, Black pepper, White pepper
Sanskrit Maricha, Vellaja, Krishna
Tamil Milagoo, Milaagu, Yavanappiriyam
Botanical Piper nigrum

As India is a major producer of good quality pepper, Indians use pepper in abundance in their daily lives. While black pepper is obtained by drying unripe green pepper berries in the sun until they turn black, white peppercorns are obtained from pepper berries which are allowed to fully ripen on the vine to a red colour before they are shelled to reveal the white peppers within.

Pepper has an aromatic and pungent flavour, and whole peppercorns keep their flavour indefinitely. As freshly ground pepper is vastly superior in flavour to its ready-ground counterpart, it is best to store whole peppercorns and grind them just before use. Peppercorns should be kept in airtight containers, away from sunlight. Pepper is widely used in Indian savoury dishes and are commonly added to marinades for meat and chicken.

Black pepper helps in digestion and also serves as an appetite stimulant. South Indians often serve *rasam*, a thin, spicy soup made with tamarind and pepper just before or after a meal to enhance appetites or aid digestion. For many South Indians who are vegetarians, consuming lentils as a source of protein may lead to excessive flatulence; this is often counteracted by drinking rasam. Other traditional treatments using pepper include remedies for coughs, colds, fever, asthma and constipation.

A paste of ground pepper is also used as an ointment to relieve skin irritations such as hives. In India, some organic agriculturists use ground pepper mixed with water to spray on plants as a natural insecticide. The same solution can also be sprinkled on areas infested with ants.

Fever Remedy

Holy basil leaves 15
Black peppercorns ¹/₂ tsp
Grated jaggery 3 tsp
Hot water 150 ml (5 fl oz / ⁵/₈ cup)

Using mortar and pestle, pound basil leaves, peppercorns and jaggery together into a coarse mixture.

Add water, stir well and steep for 1–2 minutes, then strain liquid and drink.

Anti-flatulence Remedy

Ground black pepper ¹/₂ tsp
Ground cumin ¹/₂ tsp
Ground ginger ¹/₂ tsp
Warm water 250 ml (8 fl oz / 1 cup)

Mix all ingredients together into a drink when necessary.

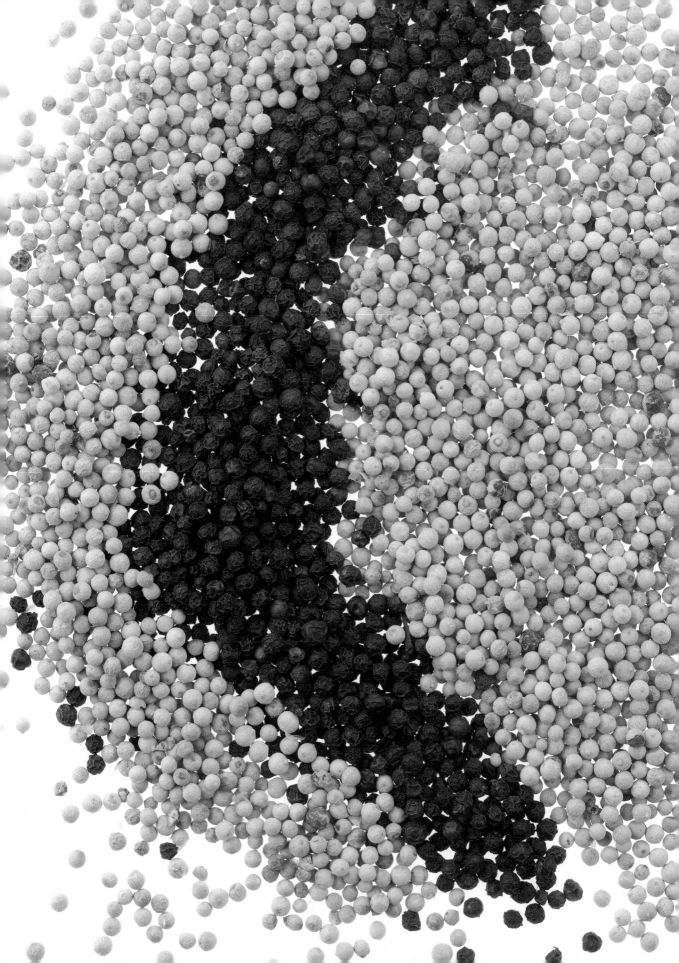

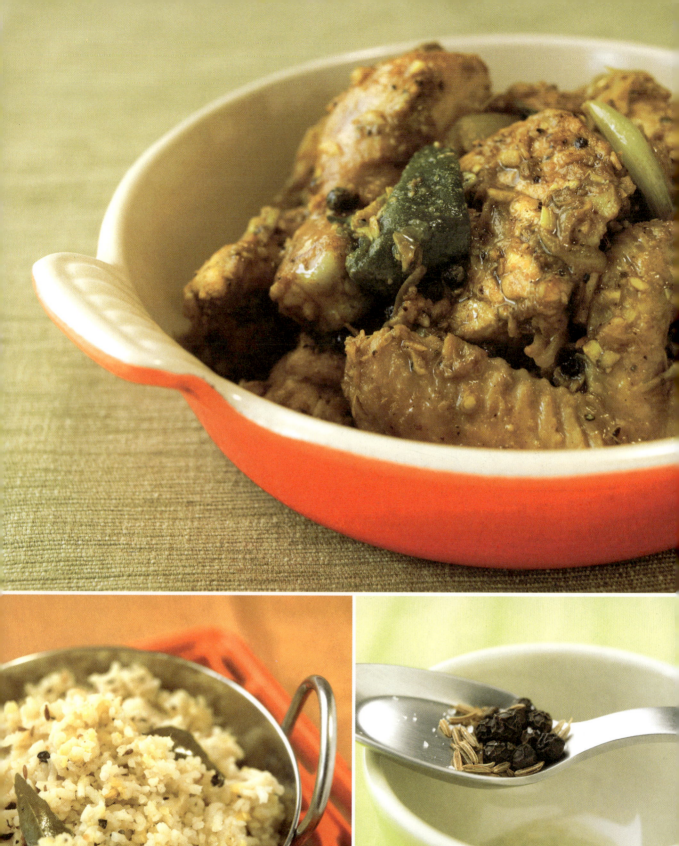
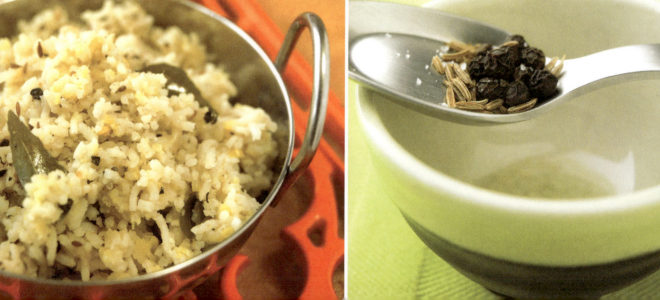

Black Pepper Chicken

Preparation time: 15 minutes
Cooking time: 15 minutes
Serves: 6

Cooking oil 3 Tbsp

Cinnamon stick 1, about 4-cm (2-in) long

Cardamoms 5

Cloves 5

Fennel seeds 1 tsp, coarsely pounded

Black peppercorns $1^1/_2$ tsp

Onions 2, medium, peeled and finely chopped

Green chillies 4, slit lengthwise

Ginger 2-cm (1-in) knob, peeled and sliced

Garlic 6 cloves, peeled and sliced

Curry leaves 2 sprigs, stems discarded

Chicken $1^1/_2$ kg (3 lb $4^1/_2$ oz), skinned and chopped into pieces

Coriander (cilantro) powder 2 tsp

Garam masala 2 tsp

Salt $1^1/_4$ tsp

Freshly ground black pepper $1^1/_4$ tsp

Heat oil and fry cinnamon, cardamoms, cloves, fennel seeds and peppercorns until aromatic.

Add onions, chillies, ginger, garlic and curry leaves and sauté until onions turn golden brown.

Add remaining ingredients except pepper and cook, stirring occasionally, until chicken is cooked.

Add pepper and cook, stirring over high heat until gravy is thick and almost dry, and chicken-pieces are well-coated with gravy. Serve hot with rice and other dishes.

Pepper Rice

Preparation time: 15 minutes
Cooking time: 15 minutes
Serves: 6

Ghee (clarified butter) 2 Tbsp

Cumin seeds 1 Tbsp

Ginger 4-cm (2-in) knob, peeled and minced

Black peppercorns $1^1/_2$ Tbsp, coarsely pounded

Curry leaves 2 sprigs, stems discarded

Rice 500 g (1 lb $1^1/_2$ oz), washed and drained

Skinned split green (mung) beans (*moong* dhal) 150 g ($5^1/_3$ oz), washed and drained

Water 1.5 litres (48 fl oz / 6 cups)

Salt $1^3/_4$ tsp

Heat ghee and fry cumin seeds until aromatic. Add ginger, pounded peppercorns and curry leaves and sauté until aromatic.

Transfer fried mixture to the rice cooker and add remaining ingredients. Stir to mix well and switch on rice cooker.

When rice is cooked, serve with any meat or vegetable dish.

Cough Reliever

This remedy is great for relieving coughs and sore throats.

Black peppercorns $^1/_4$ tsp

Salt a pinch

Caraway seeds a pinch

Mix all ingredients together and suck on mixture until it disintegrates.

Pomegranate

The pomegranate is a roundish fruit which is crowned with a prominent calyx at the bottom. The tough, leathery skin typically ranges in colour from yellow tinged with different shades of pink to a brilliant red. The inside of the fruit is separated by white, spongy tissue into compartments and packed full of juicy sacs filled with seeds.

Pomegranates are either very sweet, or sweet and sour at the same time. While the sweet varieties are best eaten fresh, the sweet and sour seeds can be sun-dried and used as a spice known as *anardhana* to add a tangy flavour to North Indian food.

All parts of the pomegranate plant including the roots, bark, leaves, flowers and fruit are used in traditional Indian healing. Ancient medical texts in India have documented the fruit as an easily digestible food that is a tonic for the heart; the sweet and sour varieties also reduce inflammation of the stomach lining and relieves heartburn. The juice from the fresh fruit is a cooling drink which helps relieve the thirst of those down with fever. Pomegranate juice also acts on the liver and kidneys to strengthen their functions; it helps to build up the body's resistance against viral infections.

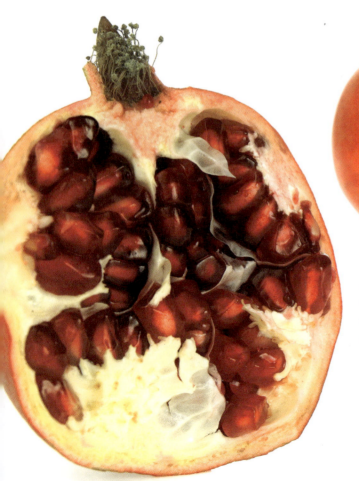

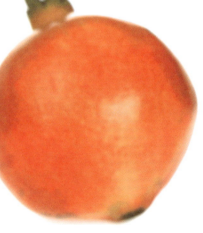

Common Pomegranate
Sanskrit Dadima, Darimba, Madhubiija
Tamil Mandulai, Mandulam
Botanical Punica granatum

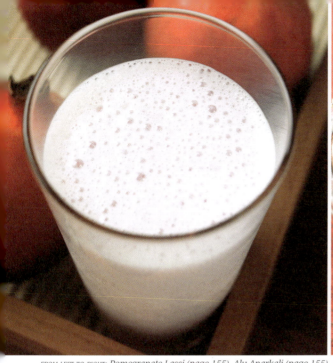
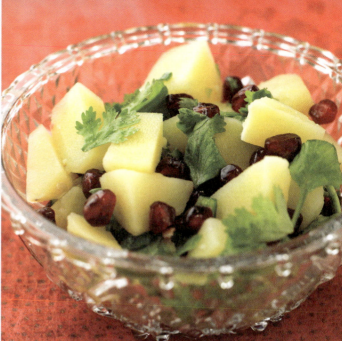

FROM LEFT TO RIGHT: Pomegranate Lassi (page 155), Alu Anarkali (page 155)

Pomegranate Lassi

Preparation time: 10 minutes
Serves: 3

Freshly squeezed pomegranate juice 200 ml (6²/₃ fl oz / ³/₄ cup)

Natural yoghurt 200 ml (6²/₃ fl oz / ³/₄ cup)

Milk 300 ml (10 fl oz /1¹/₄ cups)

Ginger juice 1 Tbsp

Honey 2–3 Tbsp

Ice cubes 9–10, standard-sized

Blend (process) all ingredients together in a blender (processor) until frothy. Serve this drink immediately.

Alu Anarkali

Preparation time: 15 minutes
Cooking time: 15 minutes
Serves: 5

Pomegranate 1, seeds removed and reserved for use

Potatoes 500 g (1 lb 1¹/₂ oz), boiled, peeled and cut into 1-cm (¹/₂- in) cubes

Chopped mint leaves 2 Tbsp

Chopped coriander (cilantro) leaves 2 Tbsp

Salad Dressing

Lime juice 100 ml (3¹/₃ fl oz / ³/₈ cup)

Grated jaggery 1¹/₂ Tbsp

Salt 1 tsp

Green chillies 2, finely chopped

Combine ingredients for salad dressing and stir well to dissolve jaggery and salt.

Put pomegranate seeds and potato cubes into a salad bowl. Pour prepared salad dressing over and toss gently to combine.

Sprinkle with chopped mint and coriander leaves. Serve immediately as an appetiser, or with rice and other dishes.

155

Rice

Common Rice, Asian rice, Common rice, Paddy rice
Sanskrit Vrihi
Tamil Pacharisi, Risi
Botanical Oryza sativa

Rice plays a very important role in Indian culture. A symbol of prosperity and fertility, rice is featured in many sacred Hindu ceremonies such as weddings.

In Indian cooking, basmati rice, a long-grain, fragrant white rice, is commonly used. Old rice is preferred over new rice as the rice grains tend to be more fluffy when cooked, even when too much water is added. In Indian cuisine, rice is usually served with curries or made into sweet or savoury snacks. South Indians often serve porridge, cooked with short, broken rice grains to the sick and the old as it can be easily digested.

A good source of B vitamins, such as thiamin and niacin, rice has only a trace of fat and and is both sodium and gluten-free. As rice has a low fibre content, it is gentle on the digestive system. When cooked with ingredients such as milk, nuts and saffron, rice serves as a very good source of energy for the body. It is also used in many beauty treatments as it is known to make the skin smooth and soft. In rural India, the womenfolk would often reserve the water from rice-washing for bathing, in order to achieve a clear and soft skin.

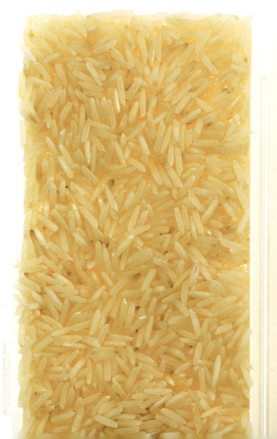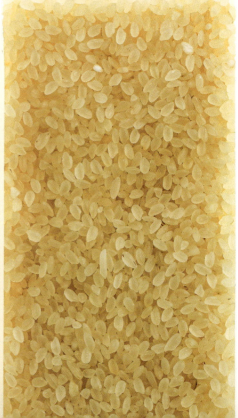

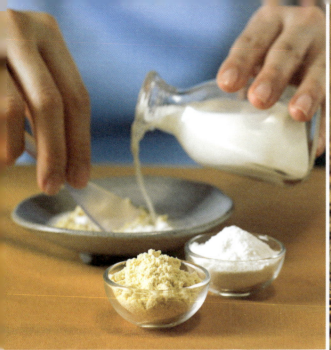
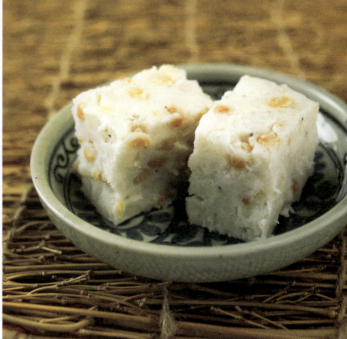

FROM LEFT TO RIGHT: *Facial Scrub (page 157), Venna Puttu (page 157)*

Facial Scrub

Rice flour 2 Tbsp
Chickpea flour (*besan*) 1 Tbsp
Milk 3 Tbsp

Combine all ingredients and use mixture immediately to scrub face and body.

Rinse off with tepid water.

Venna Puttu

Preparation time: 15 minutes
Cooking time: 15 minutes
Serves: 8

Split dried chickpeas (*channa* dhal) 120 g (4^1/$_2$ oz)
Rice flour 500 g (1 lb 1^1/$_2$ oz)
Thick coconut milk 900 ml (28^1/$_2$ fl oz / 3^5/$_8$ cups) (see page 50)
Screwpine (pandan) leaves 5, tied into a knot
Water 250 ml (8 fl oz / 1 cup)
Sugar 300 g (10^1/$_2$ oz)
Salt ^{1}/$_2$ tsp
Cardamon powder ^{1}/$_2$ tsp
Ghee (clarified butter) 2 tsp

Wash chickpeas thoroughly and boil in enough water to cover for 45 minutes, or until cooked but still firm. Drain and set aside.

Dry-roast rice flour until aromatic, sieve into a mixing bowl and set aside to cool thoroughly.

When cool, add coconut milk and stir to form a lump-free batter.

In a separate pan, boil screwpine leaves, water, sugar and salt until sugar dissolves. Reduce heat to low and discard screwpine leaves.

Slowly pour prepared batter into simmering sugar mixture while stirring constantly, until mixture thickens.

Remove from heat and stir in chickpeas, cardamom powder and ghee. Combine well.

Spread mixture into a greased 20-cm (10-in) square cake tin. Leave to set. When rice-flour cake is firm, cut into slices of desired size and serve as a snack.

Saffron

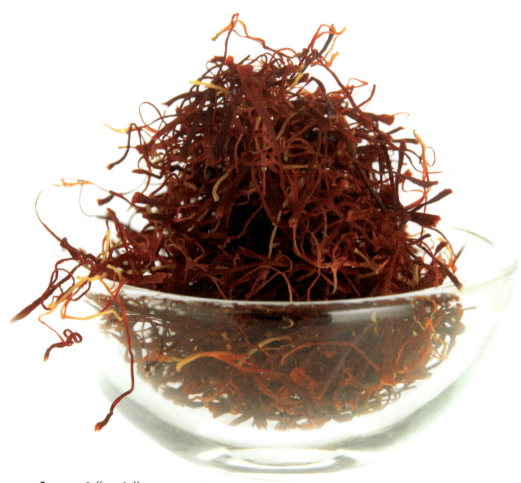

Common Saffron, Saffron crocus
Sanskrit Kumkuma, Kashmira
Tamil Klungumapu, Kungumapu
Botanical Crocus sativus

The world's most expensive spice, saffron are the stigmas of a flowering plant belonging to the crocus family. Its exorbitant price is due to the fact that at least 225,000 stigmas must be hand-picked just to produce one pound of the spice. Often dubbed as 'the golden spice', the delicate, thread-like spice has a distinctive aroma and a rather bitter flavour.

In Indian cooking, saffron is used in quite a lot of festive dishes like briyanis and rich desserts. When using saffron threads, place the strands in a clean and dry frying pan and lightly toast over very low heat for about 30 seconds only or until aromatic. Be very careful not to burn the threads. When cool, simply crush finely and use as required.

As a spice with medicinal properties, saffron improves digestion and acts as an appetite stimulant. It also soothes other stomach disorders including colic and cramps. Saffron milk is a flavourful, soothing drink that is helpful in relieving chest pains. It is also believed that saffron, when taken in small quantities, helps to regulate the menstrual cycle and relieve mentrual cramps.

Saffron is also used to treat fevers and calm nerves. As saffron has antiseptic properties, rubbing sore gums with the spice can reduce inflammation and relieve pain. To apply, crush a few threads of saffron into a powder, then dab some powder onto a finger and gently massage gums with powder.

Flu Remedy for Babies

Saffron 10 strands
Milk 1 Tbsp

Heat saffron and milk together in a metal spoon over low heat to obtain a paste. Let cool to room temperature.

When cool, apply paste on the forehead of the baby when baby is sleeping at night. Let the paste dry and wash off in the morning.

Royal Saffron Mask

This mask has many benefits. It smoothens fatigue lines and delays wrinkles, stimulates blood circulation resulting in a golden glow, soothes tension, helps to remove dark circles under the eyes and sloughs off dead skin cells.

Chickpea flour (*besan*) 1 Tbsp
Ground almond 1 Tbs
Saffron 10 strands
Sandalwood powder 1 tsp
Lukewarm milk 60 ml (2 fl oz / 1/4 cup)

Put all ingredients into a small mixing bowl and stir to combine well.

Spread a thin layer of paste on clean and dry face, avoiding the eye contours.

Leave on for about 15 minutes or until well-dried.

Rinse off thoroughly and pat dry with a clean towel.

When it comes to beauty, saffron is one of the most valuable natural beauty aids available. During the olden days, it was used to keep pimples at bay and soothe a rash. It was known to impart smoothness to a woman's skin and also give her complexion a golden tint. The spice was so desirable that even pregnant women drank saffron-infused milk in the hope that their unborn babies would acquire a golden complexion. Due to the efficacy of the spice in beauty treatments, the use of saffron in the cosmetic industry is now fairly widespread.

Saffron Kheer

Preparation time: 30 minutes
Cooking time: 10 minutes
Serves: 4

Almonds 80 g (3 oz), blanched

Rice grains 30 g (1 oz), soaked
for 30 minutes

Milk 1.25 litres (40 fl oz / 5 cups)

Saffron a generous pinch

Caster (superfine) sugar 80 g (3 oz)

Cardamom powder $^1/_2$ tsp

Blend (process) almonds, rice grains and 250 ml (8 fl oz / 1 cup) milk in a blender (processor) until smooth.

Meanwhile, bring remaining milk with saffron to the boil, then reduce heat and simmer until milk takes on the colour of saffron.

Pour in blended ingredients and stir constantly until mixture thickens.

Stir in sugar and cardamom powder and simmer until sugar dissolves. Serve warm or cold as a dessert.

Saffron Pineapple Halwa

Preparation time: 20 minutes
Cooking time: 10 minutes
Serves: 5

Melted ghee (clarified butter)
100 ml ($3^1/_2$ fl oz / $^3/_8$ cup)

Semolina 220 g (8 oz)

**Water and reserved syrup from
canned pineapple** 650 ml
(20 fl oz / $2^1/_2$ cups)

Saffron strands 10 strands

Salt $^1/_4$ tsp

Caster (superfine) sugar 200 g (7 oz)

Cardamoms 12, pounded

Cashew nuts 80 g (3 oz), chopped and
fried in ghee (clarified butter)

Raisins 80 g (3 oz), fried in ghee
(clarified butter)

Canned pineapple 300 g ($10^1/_2$ oz),
coarsely chopped

Heat ghee and lightly fry semolina until fragrant.

Meanwhile, bring water and syrup mixture to the boil with saffron strands and salt.

Pour syrup mixture with semolina into non-stick pan and stir constantly over low heat until mixture becomes a thick paste.

Stir in remaining ingredients and combine well.

Spoon halwa into a greased tray and spread out evenly. Allow to cool before scooping serving portions onto small plates to serve as a dessert.

Note: If halwa with a firmer texture is preferred, refrigerate to set for a few hours before cutting into desired shapes to serve.

Saffron-Infused Milk

A daily drink of saffron-infused milk for a period of time enables the body to build up resistance against some common ailments such as the common cold and asthma. Taking this remedy 2–3 times a day also helps relieve menstrual cramps.

Saffron a few strands

Milk 250 ml (8 fl oz / 1 cup)

Sugar 1 Tbsp

Bring all ingredients to the boil together. Remove from heat and let saffron strands infuse for a few minutes before drinking.

CLOCKWISE FROM TOP: Saffron Pineapple Halwa (page 160), Royal Saffron Mask (page 159), Saffron Kheer (page 160)

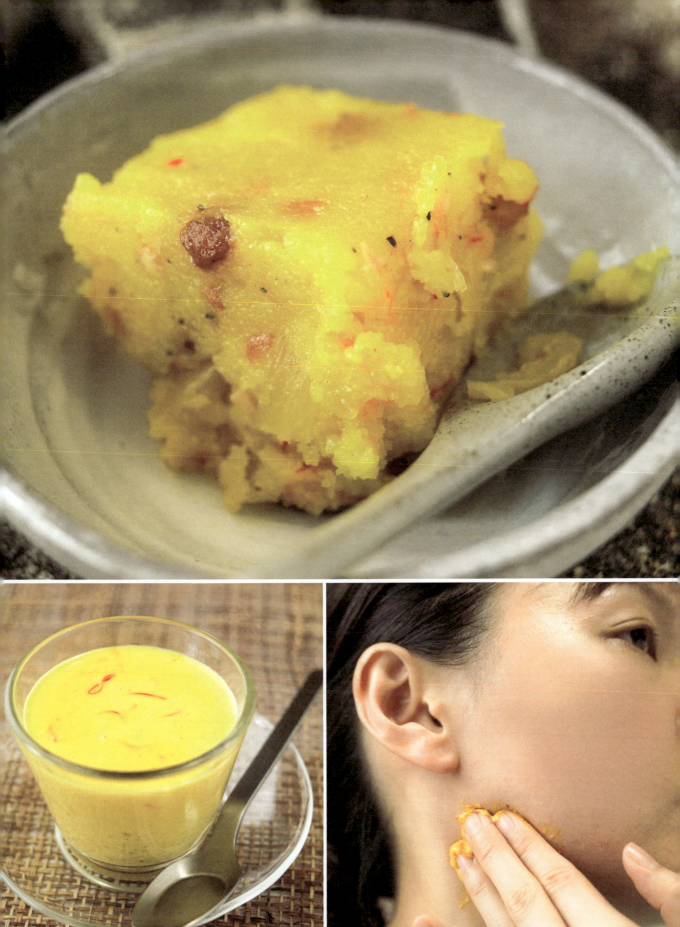

Sandalwood

Common Sandalwood, Indian sandalwood, White sandalwood

Sanskrit Chandanah, Ananditam, Tarliaparnam

Tamil Sandanam, Santhanam, Ven santhanum

Botanical Santalum album

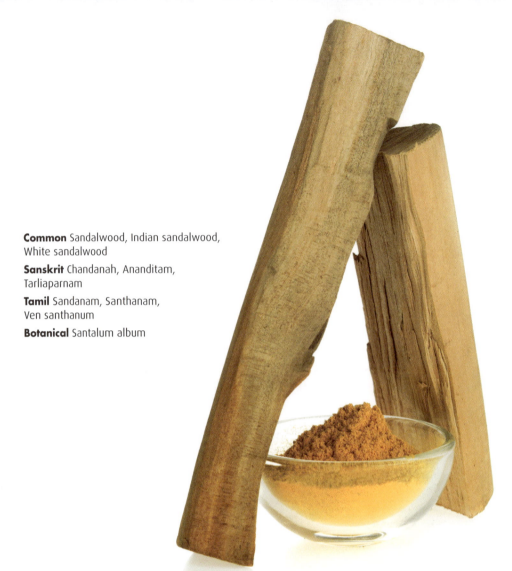

Sandalwood, also known as white sandalwood, is a very aromatic wood that is used for perfumery throughout the world. The essential oil is concentrated in the heartwood of the evergreen tree cultivated mainly in South India.

Although another variety of sandalwood known as red sandalwood (*Santalum rubrum*) is also cultivated in India, this variety is solely used for producing a natural dye. The sandal tree is very highly revered in Hinduism as well as in traditional Indian medicine. The fragrant scent of sandalwood is said to have a calming effect on the mind and helps relieve tension and anxiety when used as an oil in aromatherapy or in incense and perfumes. Traditionally, the wood, which is known to have antiseptic properties, is ground with water into a paste and applied topically on skin rash, insect bites, prickly heat areas and acne. It also has mild analgesic properties and is believed to be effective in relieving minor chest and abdominal pains. Used also as a 'cooling' agent, sandalwood paste is applied on the forehead to bring down fever or mixed with coconut juice and drunk. Known for its anti-inflammatory properties, sandalwood powder mixed with rose water and applied on the face, acts as an anti-ageing agent by protecting the skin from sun damage.

Acne Mask

White sandalwood powder 2 tsp
Rose petal powder 1 tsp
Neem powder 1 tsp
Turmeric powder 1/4 tsp
Lime juice 1 Tbsp
Water 1 Tbsp

Mix all ingredients into a paste and apply all over clean face, avoiding the eye and mouth areas.

Leave on for 20 minutes, then rinse off thoroughly and pat dry with a clean towel.

Note: Apply this treatment at night just before going to bed. Do not apply any night cream or facial moisturiser after completing treatment.

Anti-wrinkle Mask

Pure sandalwood oil 3 drops
Honey 2 tsp
Milk 1 Tbsp
Egg white 1

Mix all ingredients together and whisk lightly with a fork to form an emulsion.

Brush mixture all over clean face and neck, avoiding the eye and mouth areas.

Leave on to dry completely for 10–20 minutes, then rinse off with cool water thoroughly and pat dry with a clean towel.

Anti-Blemish Scrub

White sandalwood powder 60 g (2 oz)
Rice flour 2 tsp
Milk 50 ml (1²/₃ fl oz / 1/4 cup)
Rose water 1 Tbsp

Mix all ingredients into a paste.

Scrub all over damp face and body in a gentle circular motion for a few minutes.

Rinse off thoroughly and pat dry with a clean towel.

Note: Use this scrub 3 times a week to achieve an unblemished, smooth and supple skin.

FROM LEFT TO RIGHT: Anti-wrinkle Mask (page 163), Acne Mask (page 163)

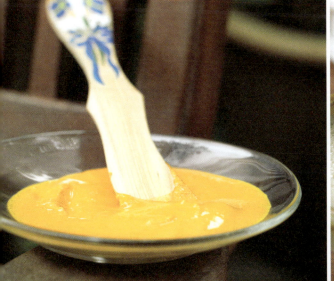
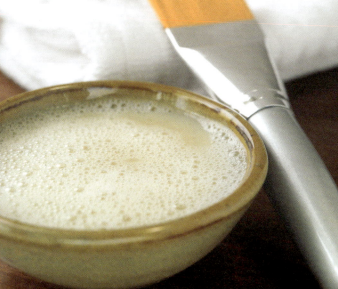

Common Sesame, White Sesame, Gingelly
Sanskrit Tila
Tamil Ellu, Illu
Botanical Sesamum indicum

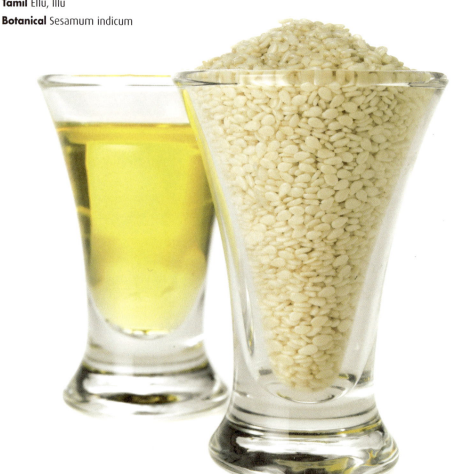

The flat, teardrop-shaped sesame seed is ivory white in colour when hulled. When eaten raw, sesame seeds taste delicately sweet and nutty. When toasted, the seeds taste like roasted peanuts. Rich in vitamins B and E as well as calcium and iron, raw sesame seeds are ground to produce a pale yellow oil, also known as gingelly oil, which has been used as a healthy cooking medium in some parts of India since ancient times. Sesame seeds which have undergone the oil-press treatment and referred to as 'seed cakes', are rich in protein and therefore often eaten, mixed with a bit of jaggery or added to stir-fries.

Gingelly oil has also been used in natural remedies, especially as a massage oil in Ayurvedic healing for centuries. Gingelly oil has emollient properties and is believed to be 'cooling' and therefore calming for the body. In beauty treatments, gingelly oil is often added to natural masks for its wrinkle-free benefits. Its antiseptic properties make sesame oil a good ointment to soothe a minor burn or sunburn as well as to speed up the healing process. The seeds can be ground and mixed with water to make poultices for healing minor skin irritations. With its high vitamin E content, gingelly oil used in cooking is also beneficial for the heart and nervous system.

Medicinally, sesame seeds are mildly laxative; eating them helps relieve constipation and remove worms from the intestinal tract. An aid to digestion, sesame seeds can stimulate blood circulation and are used for the treatment of menstrual disorders. It is believed that eating a teaspoonful of ground sesame seeds twice daily will help to regulate the menstrual cycle as well as prevent menstrual cramps.

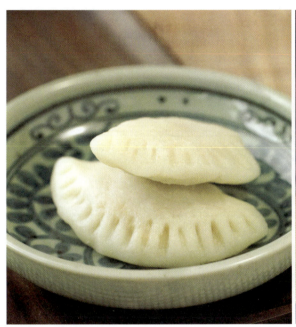 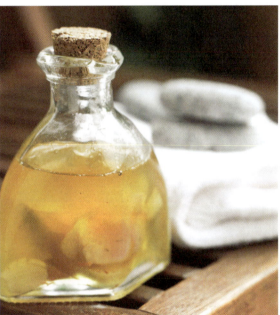

FROM LEFT TO RIGHT: Ellu Khozhakattai (page 167), Gingelly Massage Oil (page 165)

Gingelly Massage Oil

This massage oil is good for removing 'wind' from the body.

Shallots 4, peeled
Ginger 2 peeled slices
Gingelly oil 200 ml ($6^2/_3$ fl oz / $^3/_4$ cup)

Using mortar and pestle, pound shallots and ginger together coarsely.

Bring pounded ingredients to the boil with oil and remove from heat immediately.

Cool oil to lukewarm temperature before massaging onto body.

Leave on for 20 minutes then wipe off with a clean towel. Do not shower until about 5 hours later to allow treatment to fully take effect.

Note: This massage oil can be kept for up to a week at room temperature.

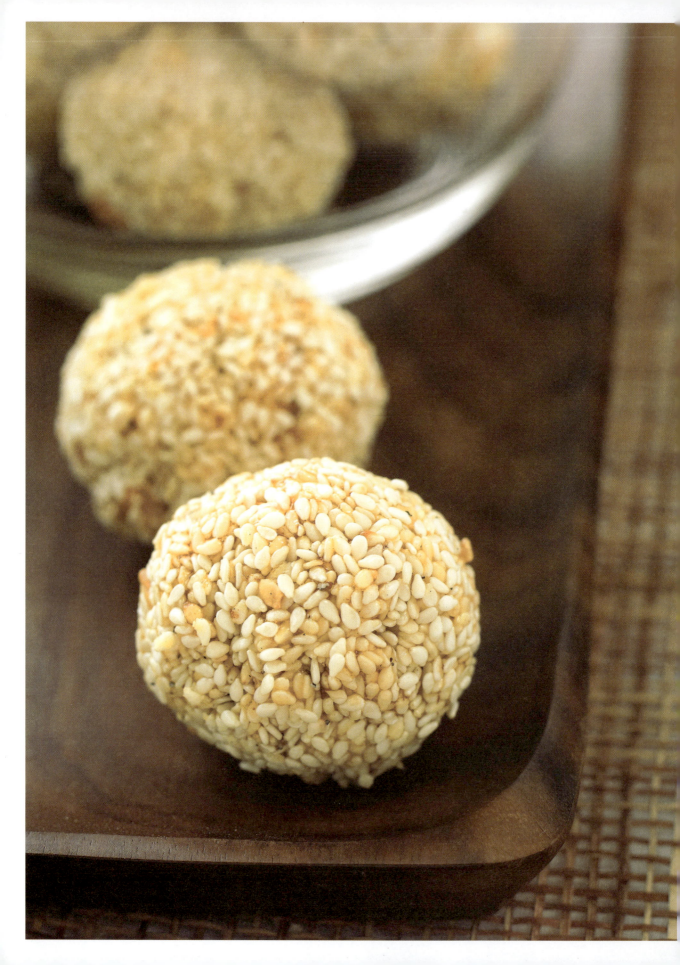

Ellu Khozhakattai (Rice Dumplings with Sesame Filling)

Water 1 litre (32 fl oz / 4 cups)

Cooking oil 2 Tbsp

Salt 1 tsp

Rice flour 500 g (1 lb 1¹/₂ oz)

Filling

White sesame seeds 230 g (8 oz)

Chopped jaggery 300 g (10¹/₂ oz)

Cardamom powder 1 tsp

Ginger powder 1 tsp

Melted ghee (clarified butter) 3 Tbsp

Prepare filling. Dry-roast sesame seeds until light brown. Grind with jaggery to form a coarse mixture. Place in a mixing bowl. Add remaining ingredients and stir to combine well.

Bring water to the boil with oil and salt, then reduce heat and simmer. Add rice flour while water is simmering and stir vigorously until a thick paste is formed. Remove from heat and knead well.

Divide dough into lime-sized balls. Take a ball of dough and with greased palms, pat into a disc. Put 2 tsp filling on one half of a disc, then fold over other half to enclose filling. Press edges well with the tines of a fork to seal. Place dumpling on a greased steaming tray.

Repeat until all ingredients are used up. Steam for 5 minutes or until cooked. Serve hot or warm as a dessert or snack.

Arthritis Rub

Red chilli 1, seeded

Ginger 2-cm (1-in) knob, peeled

Gingelly oil 250 ml (8 fl oz / 1 cup)

Using mortar and pestle, pound chilli and ginger together coarsely.

Simmer pounded ingredients in oil for 5 minutes.

Cool completely and strain into a sterilised glass bottle.

Use oil to rub and massage affected areas when necessary.

Note: This massage oil can be kept for up to a week at room temperature.

Sesame Laddu

Preparation time: 25 minutes
Cooking time: 15 minutes
Makes: 25

White sesame seeds 560 g (1 lb 3¹/₂ oz)

Ghee (clarified butter) 2 Tbsp

Coconut flesh 120 g (4¹/₂ oz), cut into pieces

Water 150 ml (5 fl oz / ⁵/₈ cup)

Chopped jaggery 360 g (12¹/₂ oz)

Caster (superfine) sugar 100 g (3¹/₂ oz)

Ginger powder 2 tsp

Cardamom powder 1 tsp

Salt a pinch

In a heavy-based saucepan, dry-roast sesame seeds until light brown and set aside.

Heat ghee and fry coconut until lightly browned. Set aside.

Prepare syrup by boiling water, jaggery and caster sugar together in a heavy-based pan over low heat until syrup turns thick and sticky.

Add sesame seeds, coconut pieces, ginger and cardamom powders and salt. Combine well and remove from heat.

While mixture is still warm, use hands to shape into small balls of desired size.

Store laddu in an airtight container and refrigerate for at least 30 minutes to obtain a firmer texture before serving as a snack or dessert.

Soap Nut

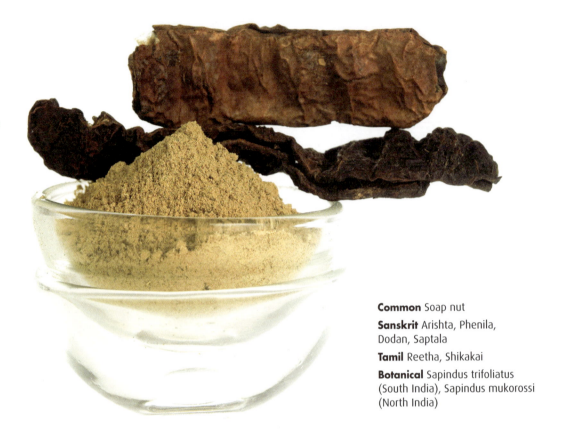

Common Soap nut

Sanskrit Arishta, Phenila, Dodan, Saptala

Tamil Reetha, Shikakai

Botanical Sapindus trifoliatus (South India), Sapindus mukorossi (North India)

Found in India and Nepal, the sun-dried fruits of the soap nut tree contain saponin, a natural cleansing agent. Soap nuts have been used in parts of India for centuries as a natural hair cleanser. The fruits are ground into a fine powder, which is mixed with water to form a paste. This paste is then applied onto hair; it lathers well and is so gentle that it does not strip hair of its natural oils, keeping hair soft and manageable. Soap nut powder is also great for cleansing oily skin without stripping the skin dry. To use, simply rub some soap nut paste all over the body and rinse off. Soap nut powder is of such a mild nature that it is even suitable for those with very sensitive skin.

During festivals such as Deepavali, the Hindus practise a ritual known as 'oil bath'; they massage their hair and bodies with gingelly or coconut oil the first thing in the morning. After about an hour, they will bathe, using soap nut powder as a cleanser. It is believed that an 'oil bath' will keep one fresh and calm for the day. In many Indian homes, soap nut is used for cleaning jewellery and gold brocade. Soap nut powder also works well as a natural, gentle laundry detergent.

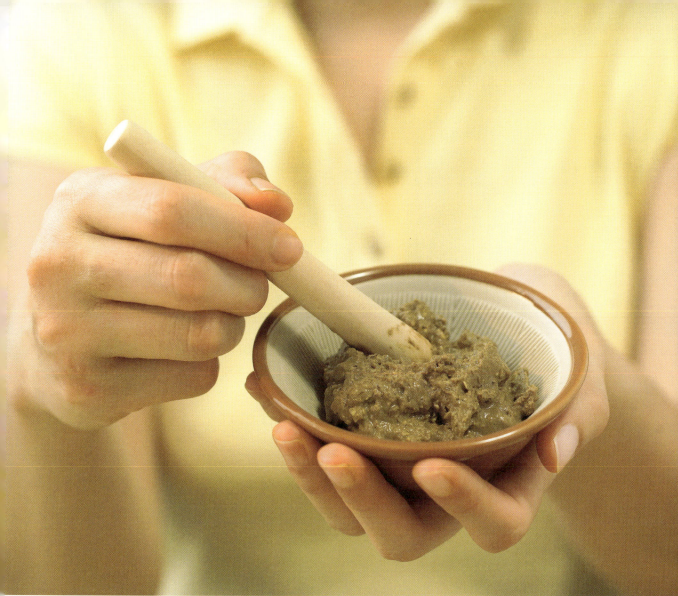

Hair Volumnising Treatment (page 169)

Hair Volumnising Treatment

Fenugreek seeds 3 Tbsp
Water 200 ml (6²/₃ fl oz / ³/₄ cup)
Soap nut powder 3 Tbsp

Soak fenugreek seeds for 6 hours. Drain and grind into a paste with water. Stir in soap nut powder to combine well.

Rub paste into scalp. Leave on for about 30 minutes, then rinse off thoroughly and shampoo as usual.

Hair Mask for Soft Hair

Use this conditioner to make your hair soft and lustrous.

Soap nut powder 50 g (2 oz)
Indian gooseberry powder 50 g (2 oz)
Freshly squeezed lemon juice 3 Tbsp
Castor oil 1 tsp
Hot water 100 ml (3¹/₃ fl oz / ³/₈ cup)

Mix all ingredients together into a paste. Apply on to damp hair.

Leave on for about 30 minutes before rinsing off. Shampoo as usual.

Tamarind

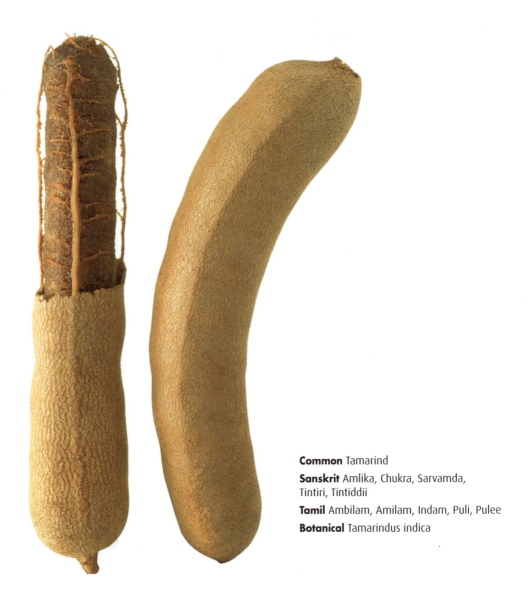

Common Tamarind
Sanskrit Amlika, Chukra, Sarvamda, Tintiri, Tintiddii
Tamil Ambilam, Amilam, Indam, Puli, Pulee
Botanical Tamarindus indica

Tamarind fruits are the sausage-shaped bean pods of a tall deciduous tree. Contained within each pod is a sticky pulp that encloses one to ten black seeds. It is the pulp that is usually used in Indian cooking as a flavouring agent for its sweet and sour taste and fruity aroma. Available as pressed brown blocks or bottled like jams, tamarind combines well with the hot-spiciness of chillies to give many South Indian dishes such as pickles and curries their hot and sour flavours and a dark brown colour.

In traditional Indian healing, tamarind preparations are available for calming fevers, curing constipation and treating stomach disorders such as gastritis and colic. Used alone, or in combination with lime juice, honey, milk, dates and spices, the pulp is known to be an effective digestive. Tamarind is also reputed to be effective in treating jaundice. In Indian folk medicine, tamarind pulp is applied topically on affected body parts to treat muscle inflammation and used in gargles for sore throats. Tamarind juice or an iced drink of tamarind syrup is also fed to persons suffering from heat stroke to help cool down their bodies.

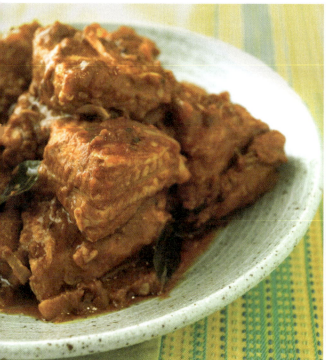 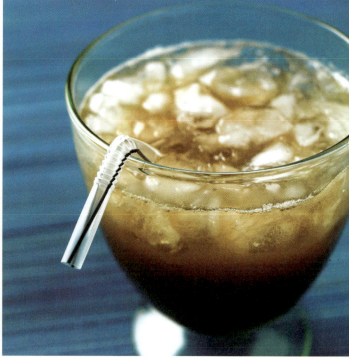

FROM LEFT TO RIGHT: Tamarind Fish (page 172), Appetite Stimulant (page 171)

Tamarind Cooler

Tamarind pulp 150 g (5^1/$_3$ oz)
Water 1.5 litres (48 fl oz / 6 cups)
Salt a pinch
Caster (superfine) sugar 150 g (5^1/$_3$ oz)

Place all ingredients in a pot and bring to boil for 10 minutes.

Strain and cool thoroughly. Serve iced as a refreshing drink.

Appetite Stimulant

Tamarind pulp 1 Tbsp

Boiling water 500 ml (16 fl oz / 2 cups)

Salt ^{1}/$_4$ tsp

Ajwain seeds 1 tsp, pounded

Mix tamarind pulp in water. Set aside to cool.

Strain liquid and stir in salt and ajwain seeds until salt dissolves. Drink as and when required.

Tamarind Rice

Preparation time: 20 minutes
Cooking time: 10 minutes
Serves: 7

Gingelly oil 250 ml (8 fl oz / 1 cup)

Cooked rice 1 kg (2 lb 3 oz), cooled

Cumin seeds 2 Tbsp

Fenugreek seeds 5 tsp

Turmeric powder 2 tsp

Chilli powder 1 tsp

Asafoetida powder 1 1/2 tsp

Split dried chickpeas (*channa* dhal)
1 1/2 Tbsp

**Skinned split black lentils
(***urad* dhal) 1 Tbsp

Black mustard seeds 1 1/2 tsp

Dried chillies 3, cut into 3-cm
(1 1/2-in) pieces

Curry leaves 3 sprigs, stems discarded

Tamarind pulp 300 ml
(10 fl oz / 1 1/4 cups), mixed with
450 ml (15 fl oz / 1 3/4 cups) water
and strained

Salt 2 1/2 tsp

Dry-roasted peanuts 100 g (3 1/2 oz)

Dry-roasted white sesame seeds
1 Tbsp

Sprinkle 50 ml gingelly oil on rice and mix well.

Dry-roast cumin and fenugreek seeds separately until aromatic and grind into a powder.

Mix ground spices with turmeric, chilli and asafoetida powders. Set aside.

Heat remaining oil and fry chickpeas and lentils until golden brown.

Add mustard seeds and dried chillies. Fry until dried chillies turn brown.

Add curry leaves and tamarind juice, then bring to the boil and simmer for 3 minutes.

Add ground spice mixture, salt and peanuts. Bring to the boil for 1 minute and remove from heat.

Pour sufficient prepared sauce over rice and mix well. Sprinkle sesame seeds on top and mix well once again. Set aside for 3 hours before serving with other dishes.

Refrigerate remaining sauce in a sterilised glass jar and use when making another batch of tamarind rice.

Note: The sauce can be stored refrigerated for up to a week.

Tamarind Stingray

Preparation time: 20 minutes
Cooking time: 15 minutes
Serves: 6

Stingray 750 g (1 lb 10 oz), cut
into large cubes

Cooking oil 3 Tbsp

Black mustard seeds 1 tsp

Cumin seeds 1 tsp

Fenugreek seeds 1 1/2 Tbsp

Onions 2, medium, peeled and
finely chopped

Garlic 10 cloves, peeled and sliced

Ginger 2-cm (1-in) knob, peeled
and sliced

Curry leaves 2 sprigs, stems discarded

Fish curry powder 5 Tbsp, mixed with
200 ml (6 2/3 fl oz / 3/4 cup) water
to form a paste

Marinade

Fish curry powder 5 Tbsp

Tamarind pulp 250 g (9 oz), mixed
with 400 ml (13 1/3 fl oz) water
and strained

Salt 1 1/2 tsp

Chopped coriander (cilantro) leaves
2 Tbsp

Mix ingredients for marinade together. Coat stingray well with marinade and set aside for 15 minutes.

Heat oil and fry mustard seeds until they stop spluttering.

Add cumin and fenugreek seeds and fry until fragrant.

Add onions, garlic, ginger and curry leaves and sauté until onions turn golden brown. Add curry paste and fry over low heat until oil separates.

Add marinated stingray and continue to simmer over low heat until cooked. Serve hot with rice and other dishes.

Tamarind Rice (page 172)

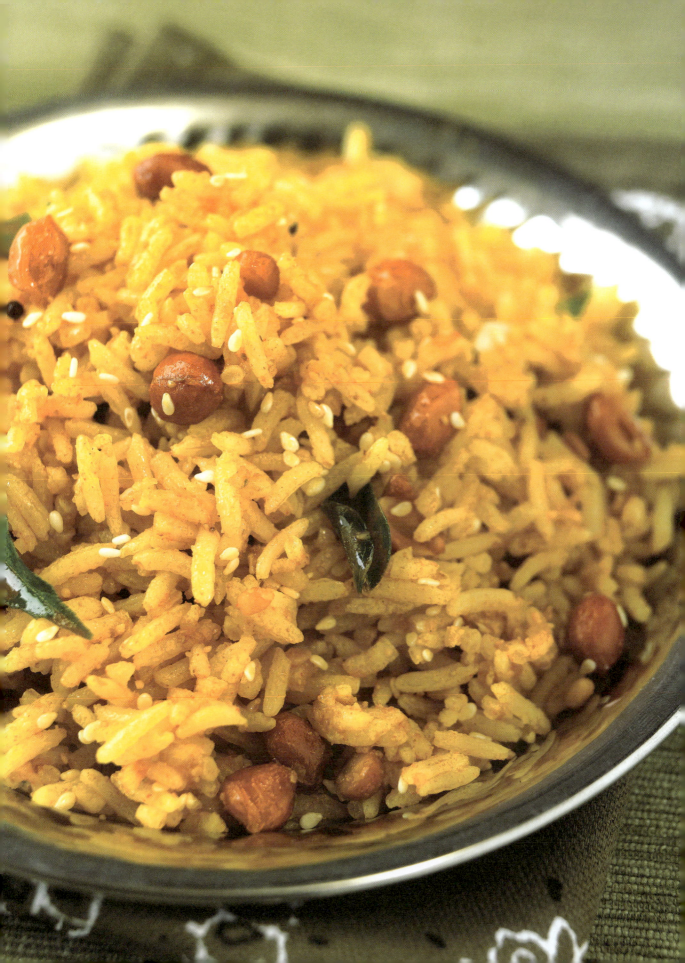

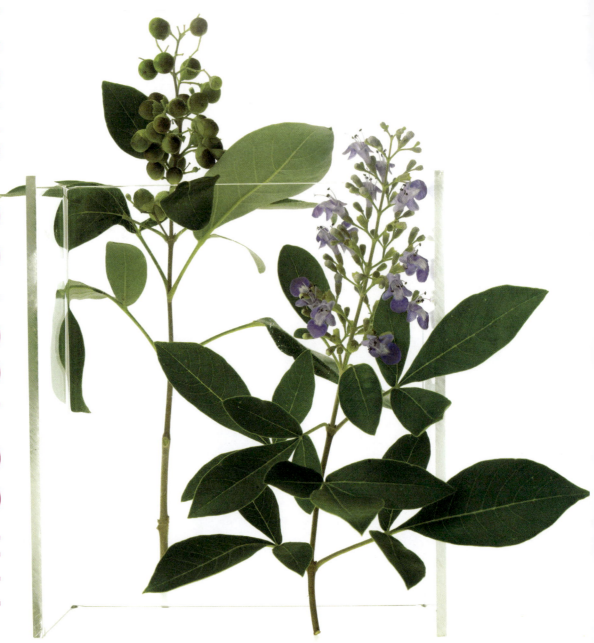

Common Three-leaved chaste tree,
Simpleleaf chaste tree
Sanskrit Jalanirgundi
Tamil Karu-nocci
Botanical Vitex trifolia

The three-leaved chaste tree is a shrubby plant; it has lance-shaped leaves which radiate from the stalks like an open hand. A very pretty tree with sprays of tiny lavender flowers, it has clusters of small berries which resemble peppercorns and, when dried, have a slight peppery aroma and flavour. While the flowers of the tree are lightly scented, its leaves and stems are rather aromatic.

While chaste leaves are often used in Indian cooking in the same way as many other green, leafy vegetables, the berries of the tree are used for a range of medicinal treatments. In fact, chaste berries are most commonly used to rectify hormonal imbalances in women who suffer from excessive levels of the female hormone, oestrogen, and insufficient levels of the other female hormone, progesterone. The regulation of the female hormones enables the female reproductive system to ovulate normally, thereby increasing the chances of pregnancy. Consequently, chaste berries are often used to treat fertility and other problems concerning the feminine reproductive system. Some traditional treatments for women include the use of chaste berries to restore absent menstruation, reduce heavy bleeding during menstruation and relieve premenstrual syndrome as well as menopausal symptoms.

Various scientific studies have shown that the regular use of remedies with chaste berries over an extended period of time may help to alleviate the symptoms of premenstrual syndrome including mood swings, bloating, migraines, cravings for sweets and the lack of mental concentration. An infusion of a teaspoonful of berries in a glass of water, to be drunk three times daily, is a commonly-prescribed remedy.

For mothers who are breastfeeding, it is believed that the use of chaste berries will also aid in increasing lactation. However, always consult your doctor or natural healer before using chaste berries for any form of medicinal treatment, especially if you are pregnant or already taking other types of hormonal drugs such as contraceptive or fertility pills.

External treatments using fresh ripe berries include a tincture produced with the pulp of the pounded fruits. This helps to relieve muscular aches and pains as well as numbness in the joints.

Remedy for Premenstrual Syndrome

Ripe chaste berries and flowers 1 tsp

Boiling water 250 ml (8 fl oz / 1 cup)

Infuse berries and flowers in water for about 15 minutes.

Drink this infusion 3 times a day, a few days before the start of, and also during, the menstrual cycle.

Herbal Chapati

Preparation time: 30 minutes
Cooking time: 10 minutes
Serves: 5

Fine wholewheat flour (*atta* flour) 500 g (1 lb 1½ oz)

Salt 1 tsp

Chaste leaves and fruits 60 g (2 oz), chopped

Finely chopped spring onion (scallion) 1 Tbsp

Finely chopped coriander (cilantro) leaves 1 Tbsp

Green chilli 1, sliced

Lukewarm water 450 ml (14 fl oz /1¾ cups)

Melted ghee (clarified butter) or cooking oil 3 Tbsp

Sift flour and salt into a large mixing bowl. Add chaste leaves and fruits, spring onion, coriander leaves and green chilli.

Add water to flour mixture gradually, mixing well and then kneading to form a stiff dough. Cover and leave aside for 30 minutes.

Knead dough again for 10 minutes or until almost elastic in texture. Divide dough into 10 equal portions. Roll into balls, then flatten into discs.

Heat a frying pan and grease lightly with melted ghee or cooking oil. Pan-fry chapati on both sides until golden brown. Repeat until all the dough is cooked.

Serve hot with curry or chutney, such as lemon and mango pickle.

Rasam with Chaste Leaves

Preparation time: 10 minutes
Cooking time: 25 minutes
Serves: 6

Skinned split green (mung) beans (*moong* dhal) 80 g (3 oz), washed and drained

Water 1.75 litres (56 fl oz / 7 cups)

Black peppercorns 1½ tsp, coarsely pounded

Cumin 2 tsp, coarsely pounded

Garlic 6 cloves, peeled and coarsely pounded

Turmeric powder 1 tsp

Chaste leaves 150 g (5⅓ oz)

Cooking oil 1½ Tbsp

Black mustard seeds 1 tsp

Dried chillies 2, cut into 2-cm (1-in) pieces

Curry leaves 2 sprigs, stems discarded

Asafoetida powder ½ tsp

Chopped coriander (cilantro) leaves 2 Tbsp

Freshly squeezed lime juice 100 ml (3⅓ fl oz / ⅜ cup)

Salt 1½ tsp

Place green beans, water, peppercorns, cumin, garlic, turmeric powder, chaste leaves and flowers in a pot and boil for 20 minutes, or until beans turn mushy.

In a separate pot, heat oil and fry mustard seeds and dried chillies until aromatic. Stir in curry leaves and asafoetida powder. Finally, add bean mixture, coriander leaves, lime juice and salt.

Bring to the boil for 1 minute and serve immediately with rice and other dishes.

CLOCKWISE FROM TOP: Herbal Chapati *(page 176),* Rasam with Chaste Leaves *(page 176),* Remedy for Premenstrual Syndrome *(page 176)*

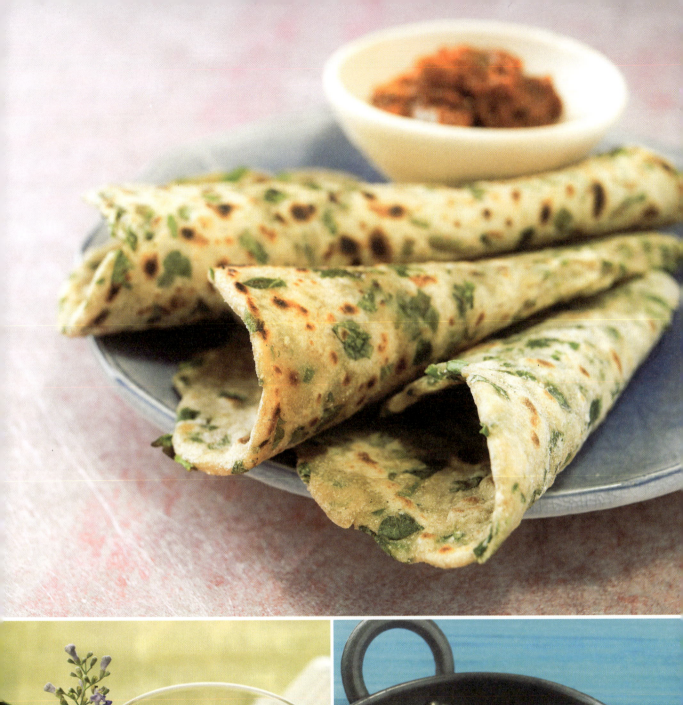

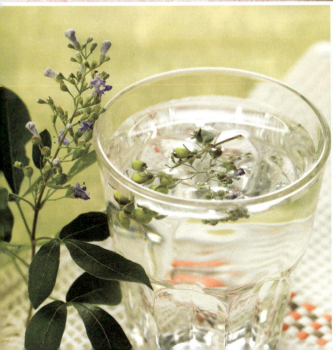

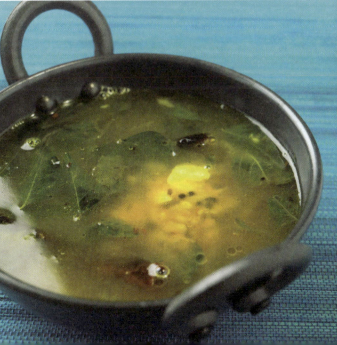

Turmeric

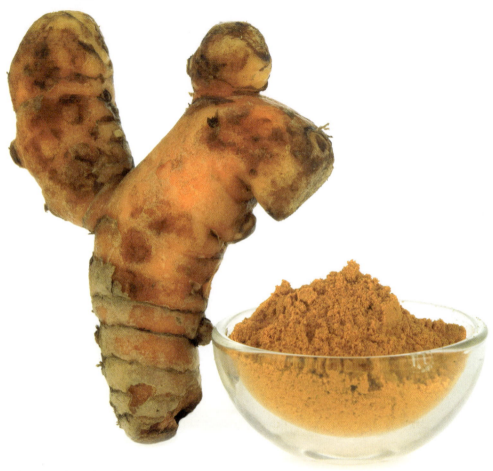

Common Turmeric, yellow ginger
Sanskrit Haridra, Marmarii, Nisha, Rajani
Tamil Manjal
Botanical Curcuma longa

The rhizome or stem of a ginger-like plant, turmeric has a segmented brown skin and bright orange flesh. Ground turmeric is made from fresh stems of turmeric which are boiled or steamed, then dried and ground into a bright yellow powder.

Mildly aromatic with a slightly earthy smell, the stem has a pungent, bitter flavour. As turmeric powder resembles saffron powder, it is often used as a cheap substitute for the latter despite the fact that both powders have very different flavours.

Due to its strong antibacterial properties, turmeric is a must-have when cooking meat or seafood as it not only helps kill bacteria but also acts as a natural preservative.

Turmeric is thus used in large amounts for making chutneys and pickles. Turmeric powder is also used in many Indian curries.

A natural pharmaceutical in itself, turmeric has been known to soothe the mucous lining of the stomach, which reduces the risk of stomach ulcers due to drugs or stress. The herb also has an anti-inflammatory effect on the cardiovascular system and regulates cholesterol in the body. Long popular as a remedy for respiratory infections such as colds, sore throats and coughs, turmeric is also used in treatments for arthritis to relieve pain and stiffness in the joints as well as for skin disorders such as acne and psoriasis. A natural antibiotic agent, turmeric is known to successfully inhibit infection whether bacterial, viral or fungal.

Turmeric Chicken Wings

Preparation time: 40 minutes
Cooking time: 15 minutes
Serves: 5

Chicken wings 750 g (1 lb 10 oz)
Turmeric powder 2 tsp
Ginger paste 2 Tbsp
Garlic paste 2 Tbsp
Meat curry powder 2 Tbsp
Chickpea flour (besan) 80 g (3 oz)
Salt 1 1/4 tsp
Cooking oil for deep-frying

Place all ingredients except cooking oil into a mixing bowl and combine well. Leave to marinate for 30 minutes.

Deep-fry chicken wings in hot oil until crispy. Drain on absorbent paper towels. Serve immediately as a snack, or with rice and other dishes.

Ointment for Burns

Pure coconut oil 2 Tbsp
Fresh aloe vera gel 2 Tbsp
Turmeric powder 1/4 tsp

Mix all ingredients together and apply on affected area.

FROM LEFT TO RIGHT: *Turmeric Chicken Wings (page 179), Ointment for Burns (page 179)*

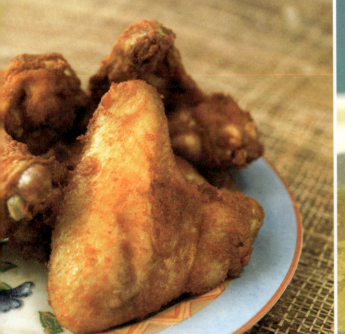
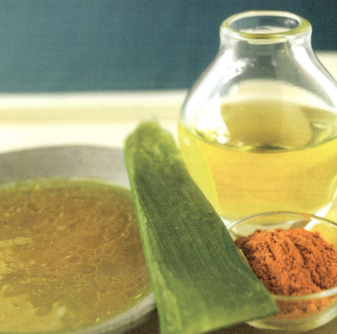

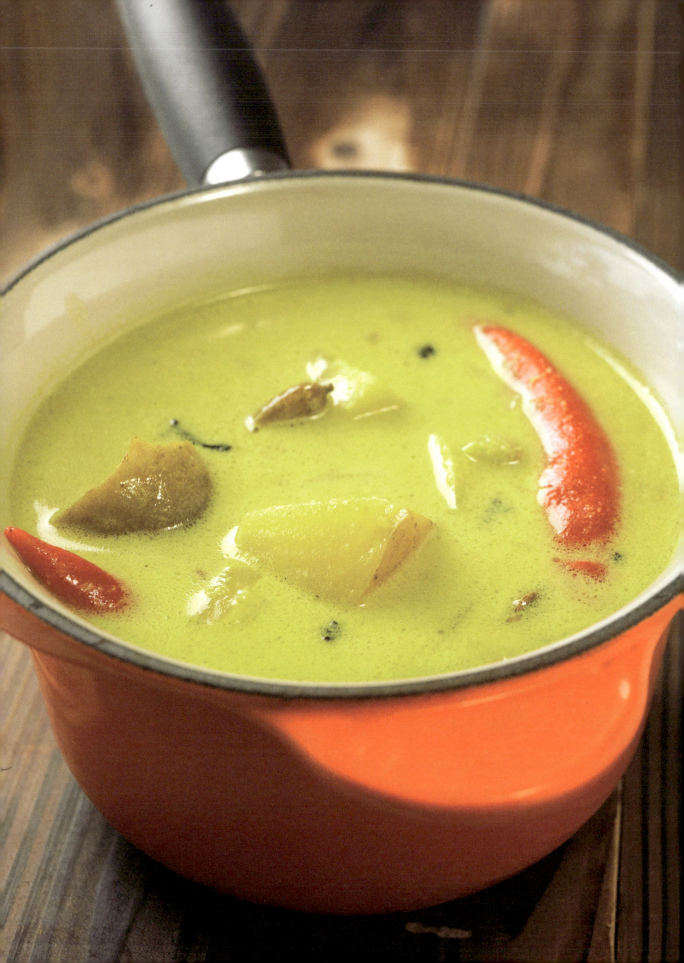

Cough Remedy

Turmeric has antiseptic properties and thus aids in curing chronic cough and throat irritation.

Fresh milk 250 ml (8 fl oz / 1 cup)

Salt a pinch

Turmeric powder 1/2 tsp

Combine milk, salt and turmeric powder together and bring to the boil over low heat.

Drink this portion at least once a day until cough subsides.

Compress for Muscle Strain or Body Ache

Turmeric powder 1 Tbsp

Ginger powder 1 Tbsp

Hot water 2 Tbsp

Mix all ingredients together into a paste.

Wrap paste in a small, clean piece of muslin cloth to form a bundle.

Press bundle on affected areas to relieve muscle strain or general body ache.

Turmeric Potato Curry

Preparation time: 15 minutes
Cooking time: 15 minutes
Serves: 6

Grated coconut 150 g (5¹/₃ oz)

Almonds 10, blanched

Red chillies 4

Ginger 2-cm (1-in) knob, peeled and left whole

Garlic 2 cloves, peeled and left whole

Turmeric powder 1¹/₂ tsp

Water 250 ml (8 fl oz / 1 cup)

Cooking oil 2 Tbsp

Onion 1, medium, peeled and sliced

Curry leaves 2 sprigs, stems discarded

Thin coconut milk 1 litre (32 fl oz / 4 cups) (see page 50)

Potatoes 800 g (1³/₄ lb), boiled and cut into cubes

Salt 1¹/₄ tsp

Thick coconut milk 250 ml (8 fl oz /1 cup) (see page 50)

Dry Spices

Cinnamon sticks 2, about 3-cm (1¹/₂-in) long each

Cardamoms 2

Cloves 4

Black mustard seeds 1 tsp

Blend (process) grated coconut, almonds, chillies, ginger, garlic, turmeric powder and water until smooth.

Heat oil and fry dry spices until aromatic.

Add onion and curry leaves and sauté until onion turns light brown.

Add blended mixture, thin coconut milk, potatoes and salt. Bring to the boil for 3 minutes, then stir in thick coconut milk. Boil for another minute while stirring constantly.

Remove from heat and serve with rice, thosai or puttu mayam.

Turmeric Potato Curry (page 181)

Winter Melon

The winter melon or ash gourd is a fruit which can grow to a weight of 5 kg for the smaller varieties, while the giant varieties can weigh up to 40 kg. Its skin is usually greyish-green in colour and its white flesh is used for cooking as well as medicinal treatments. The melon is a rich source of calcium, phosphorus, iron and vitamin C.

The Indians believe that winter melons are a 'cooling' food and therefore they usually serve them during summer time, sometimes simmered in yoghurt to make it even more 'cooling' for the hot weather. Because of its cooling properties, winter melon juice is prescribed to relieve pain from peptic ulcers. Eating winter melon regularly also helps relieve haemorrhoids as the fruit possesses laxative properties. As a diuretic, the winter melon aids in flushing out toxins from the body.

Common Winter melon, Ash gourd
Sanskrit Kushmanda
Tamil Poosanikaai
Botanical Benincasa hispida

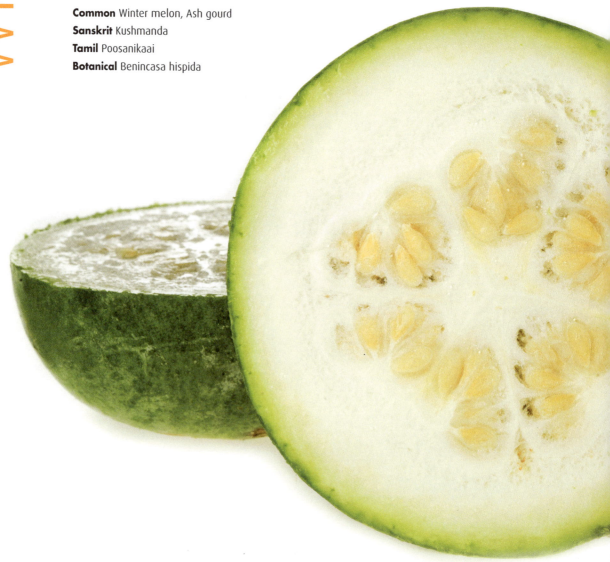

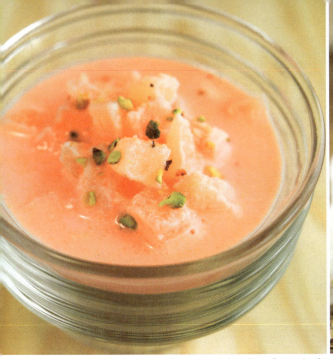
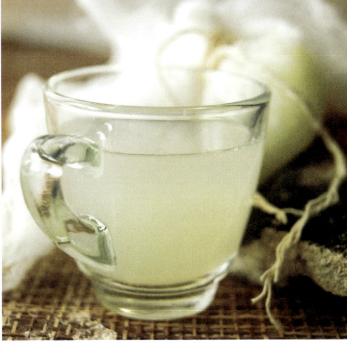

FROM LEFT TO RIGHT: Petha Chaman (page 183), Pain Reliever for Peptic Ulcers (page 183)

Petha Chaman (Candied Winter Melon Dessert)

Preparation time: 15 minutes
Cooking time: 15 minutes
Serves: 4

Full cream milk 1 litre (32 fl oz/ 4 cups)

Candied winter melon 500 g
(1 lb 1¹/₂ oz), diced

Ground almond 100 g (3¹/₂ oz)

Semolina 1 Tbsp

Rose water 1 Tbsp

Pink colouring ¹/₂ tsp

Cardamom powder ¹/₂ tsp

Pistachios 80 g (3 oz), shelled
and chopped

Put milk, winter melon, almond powder and semolina into a pot. Bring to the boil and simmer over medium heat for 10 minutes.

Add rose water, pink colouring and cardamom powder. Combine well. Serve hot or cold, sprinkled with chopped pistachios.

Pain Reliever for Peptic Ulcers

Winter melon 200g (7 oz), skinned and
left whole

Water as required

Grate winter melon and strain to extract juice.

Pour juice into a measuring cup and add an equal amount of water. Stir and drink.

Drink this portion every morning until the pain from peptic ulcers subside.

Weights and Measures

Quantities for this book are given in Metric, Imperial and American (spoon) measures. Standard spoon and cup measurements used are:
1 tsp = 5 ml, 1 Tbsp = 15 ml, 1 cup = 250 ml. All measures are level unless otherwise stated.

LIQUID AND VOLUME MEASURES

Metric	Imperial	American
5 ml	$^1/_6$ fl oz	1 teaspoon
10 ml	$^1/_3$ fl oz	1 dessertspoon
15 ml	$^1/_2$ fl oz	1 tablespoon
60 ml	2 fl oz	$^1/_4$ cup (4 tablespoons)
85 ml	$2^1/_2$ fl oz	$^1/_3$ cup
90 ml	3 fl oz	$^3/_8$ cup (6 tablespoons)
125 ml	4 fl oz	$^1/_2$ cup
180 ml	6 fl oz	$^3/_4$ cup
250 ml	8 fl oz	1 cup
300 ml	10 fl oz ($^1/_2$ pint)	$1^1/_4$ cups
375 ml	12 fl oz	$1^1/_2$ cups
435 ml	14 fl oz	$1^3/_4$ cups
500 ml	16 fl oz	2 cups
625 ml	20 fl oz (1 pint)	$2^1/_2$ cups
750 ml	24 fl oz ($1^1/_5$ pints)	3 cups
1 litre	32 fl oz ($1^3/_5$ pints)	4 cups
1.25 litres	40 fl oz (2 pints)	5 cups
1.5 litres	48 fl oz ($2^2/_5$ pints)	6 cups
2.5 litres	80 fl oz (4 pints)	10 cups

DRY MEASURES

Metric	Imperial
30 grams	1 ounce
45 grams	$1^1/_2$ ounces
55 grams	2 ounces
70 grams	$2^1/_2$ ounces
85 grams	3 ounces
100 grams	$3^1/_2$ ounces
110 grams	4 ounces
125 grams	$4^1/_2$ ounces
140 grams	5 ounces
280 grams	10 ounces
450 grams	16 ounces (1 pound)
500 grams	1 pound, $1^1/_2$ ounces
700 grams	$1^1/_2$ pounds
800 grams	$1^3/_4$ pounds
1 kilogram	2 pounds, 3 ounces
1.5 kilograms	3 pounds, $4^1/_2$ ounces
2 kilograms	4 pounds, 6 ounces

LENGTH

Metric	Imperial
0.5 cm	$^1/_4$ inch
1 cm	$^1/_2$ inch
1.5 cm	$^3/_4$ inch
2.5 cm	1 inch

OVEN TEMPERATURE

	°C	°F	Gas Regulo
Very slow	120	250	1
Slow	150	300	2
Moderately slow	160	325	3
Moderate	180	350	4
Moderately hot	190/200	370/400	5/6
Hot	210/220	410/440	6/7
Very hot	230	450	8
Super hot	250/290	475/550	9/10

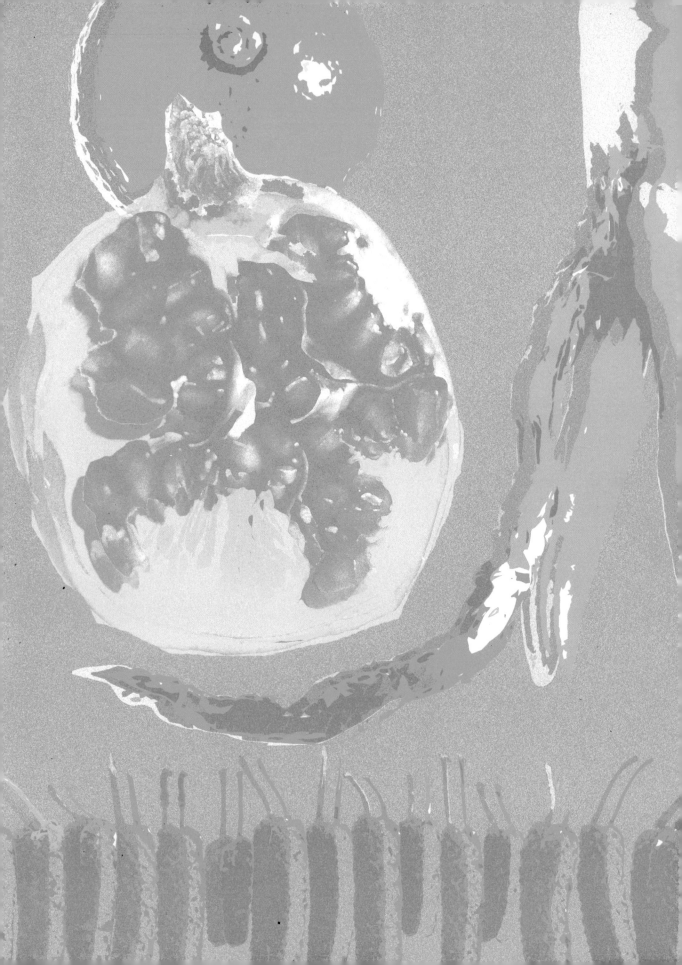